CRAIG SIMFEX

Healing from Within: A Nurse's Journey to Empower Patients

Contents

Preface

Greetings! I trust your day is off to a splendid start. How often have you heard that? Hopefully, more times than not. And, since we're all in need of a smile, here's a nursing-themed joke for you: Why can't nurses draw blood? Wait for it... They never attended art school. Okay, maybe not the funniest, but it's a start, much like my life, where comedy often writes itself.

I'm Craig, hailing from the heart of Northeast Ohio, a place known as "the mistake on the lake." Some say it's because our river famously caught fire. However, the truth lies in tycoons like Rockefeller who once used it as a convenient dumping ground for kerosene byproducts. You guessed it – gasoline. Many other companies joined in, and the Cuyahoga River managed to set itself ablaze multiple times. The true origins of this nickname, though, date back to a noble endeavor. In 1986, the United Way aimed to outdo Disneyland with a Guinness World Record for the most simultaneous balloon releases. Cleveland thought it could release 1.5 million balloons at once. Fate had other plans, and tragedy struck. For those unfamiliar, the story goes like this: the balloons were released, creating a magnificent display. However, an approaching storm forced them down during a serious search to locate two missing fishermen. Sadly, due to the sheer number of balloons in the lake, the search proved futile.

This sense of hopelessness, of being lost without a trace,

can often overwhelm us during times of illness. But take heart, for this notion is far from the truth. You can and will prevail. Spend time with me on my journey, and you'll uncover invaluable lessons, shifting your mindset and revealing your inner strength.

DISCLAIMER

The information provided in this book, titled Healing from Within: A Nurse's Journey to Empower Patients, on herbal remedies is for informational purposes only. The author, editor, and publisher assume no responsibility for the misuse of the content within this book.

Consuming any products or following the remedies outlined in this book is entirely at your own risk. The information presented makes no guarantees, expressed or implied, regarding the final results of using these remedies. It is important to note that the content in this book has not undergone review, testing, or approval by any official testing body or government agency.

Some remedies suggested in this book may not comply with FDA guidelines. The author, publisher, and editor disclaim any liability and will not be held responsible for any loss of life, injury, alleged or otherwise, that may occur directly or indirectly as a result of utilizing the information contained in this book.

Readers are advised to consult with their physician before attempting any herbal remedies mentioned in this book. This publication is not intended to be used as a medical guide, and it does not encompass all the information available on natural remedies.

By using this book, you acknowledge that you have read, understood, and agreed to the terms of this disclaimer.

ADDITIONAL DISCLAIMER

Individual Responses: The effectiveness of herbal remedies can vary from person to person. The information in this book is general and may not account for individual health conditions, allergies, or other factors that could influence the results.

Quality of Ingredients: The book may suggest the use of specific herbs or ingredients. It is essential to ensure the quality, purity, and safety of these ingredients, as variations in quality can impact the outcomes of the remedies.

No Substitute for Professional Advice: This book is not a substitute for professional medical advice, diagnosis, or treatment. Readers should not disregard, delay, or avoid seeking medical advice from qualified healthcare professionals based on information in this book.

Legal Compliance: Readers are responsible for ensuring that their use of any remedies aligns with local regulations and laws. The author, editor, and publisher do not assume responsibility for legal consequences arising from non-compliance.

Updates and Changes: Herbal knowledge evolves, and new information may emerge after the publication of this book. The author, editor, and publisher are not obligated to update the content, and readers should verify information with current sources.

Adverse Reactions: Some individuals may experience adverse reactions to herbal remedies. If you encounter any unexpected side effects, discontinue use immediately and seek medical attention.

External Resources: This book may reference external resources or websites. The author, editor, and publisher are not responsible for the content, accuracy, or availability of these external resources.

Disclaimer on Comprehensiveness: This book does not claim to encompass the entirety of herbal knowledge, and additional research from diverse sources is recommended for a comprehensive understanding of natural remedies.

Readers are urged to approach the information in this book with caution, critical thinking, and a thorough understanding of their own health circumstances.

Chapter 1: So it Begins

I n the opening chapter of our extraordinary journey, allow me to introduce myself. My name is Craig, and I've dedicated over 15 years of my life to the world of medicine, working as a compassionate Registered Nurse (RN) in various medical settings. Each day spent in the Intensive Care Unit (ICU) is a relentless battle to preserve life, but it's also a place where I've wholeheartedly embraced my role as a patient advocate.

My experiences have led me down countless hospital corridors, bringing me face to face with families in their most vulnerable moments. I've become their guide through the labyrinth of complex medical situations, and my soothing presence has often served as the calm in their storms. I've witnessed the most profound of human emotions, from the anxiety-laden hours of waiting in sterile waiting rooms to the tearful relief when a patient recovers. I've navigated the discussions surrounding end-of-life choices, holding the hands of loved ones as they made heart-wrenching decisions. The importance of advance directives, something I've often emphasized to my patients, has become a mantra in my professional life. Advance directives are legal documents that allow individuals to specify their preferences for medical treatment in the event they become unable to make medical decisions for themselves due to illness or incapacity.

As a nurse, I've had the privilege of experiencing the full spectrum of human existence. I've encountered families who, driven by fear or mistrust, choose to stay overnight in the hospital, watching over their loved ones like vigilant sentinels. The stories I have to share are a diverse collection, a rollercoaster of emotions that range from side-splitting laughter to spine-chilling terror. There have been moments that have left a permanent mark on my heart, reminders of the profound impact a nurse can have on the lives of those in their care.

We embark on a different journey, a journey where my life takes an unexpected turn, where my plans for quality family-time and a 2 week stay vacation from work are disrupted by an unforeseen adversary.

It all begins with whispers of an invisible threat that looms large over the world—a threat that will soon strike at the very heart of my existence. The name on everyone's lips, the cause of worldwide concern, is COVID-19. Little did I know that this name, which had become a constant presence in the news, would soon become a reality in my own life.

It starts with a few innocent symptoms: an upset stomach, a low-grade fever. In any other year, I might have dismissed these symptoms as a common flu. But in the era of the coronavirus, every cough and sneeze carries an ominous weight. The world's collective consciousness is gripped by fear, and the virus, like a phantom, lurks in every corner.

I make the inevitable decision to undergo the dreaded COVID-19 test. The process itself is awkward and nerve-wracking, placing me in an unfamiliar position—not as the caregiver, but as the patient. The swab, like a foreign invader, probes into the deepest recesses of my respiratory system, and the sensation is unsettling. I can't help but crack a wry smile as I contemplate the absurdity of being on the receiving end.

The relief that washes over me upon receiving a negative test result is profound, but it's a short-lived respite. With time my digestive issues worsen, a persistent reminder that something more insidious is at play.

As I take a much-needed vacation, the delicate balance between commitment and the looming threat of infection becomes real. Leading to frequent episodes of diarrhea—up to 25 times a day. The bathroom transforms into an unpredictable battleground, accompanied by cramping, bloating and persistent pain.

Leaving the safety of home becomes a daunting challenge, fueled by the fear of embarrassing accidents in public. Carrying extra underwear and pants becomes a routine necessity, a precautionary measure against the unpredictable twists of my digestive system.

Socializing turns into a battlefield of caution, where every outing is overshadowed by the fear of judgment and the uncertainty of my own body. The constant physical and mental strain takes its toll, with anxiety becoming a relentless companion, adding another layer to my already challenging struggles.

In this journey through the shadows of my own body, I grapple with the harsh reality of a life altered by persistent symptoms. As I navigate this labyrinth, my hope extends beyond physical relief to a glimpse of light in the midst of the darkness that surrounds me.

As my health declines, it becomes a test not only of my medical expertise but also of the empathy I've cultivated as a nurse. It's a journey that will take us through the depths of uncertainty, the highs of triumph, and the resilience of the human spirit. I warmly invite you to join me in reading my story, with the hope that it may offer support and guidance to you or someone you know who may be facing similar challenges.

Chapter 2: I am Damaged

I n my journey towards better health, it's not only about the serious and life-altering moments; it's also about those light-hearted exchanges that make life with my wife so delightful. I want to share one such moment, a playful interaction that occurred the day before I fell seriously ill 4 days before my covid test. It involves some tasty but suspicious onions and my wife's sense of humor.

On that day, my wife prepared a mouthwatering meal for me. It was a feast of potato and jalapeño tacos topped with a tantalizing aloe sauce. A delicious combination, indeed. However, these delectable tacos came with a surprising twist – they were garnished with purple onions.

As we sat down to enjoy this delightful meal, I couldn't resist making a wisecrack about the onions. You see, there had recently been a recall on onions due to a salmonella outbreak. So, with a twinkle in my eye, I jokingly told my wife that she was trying to poison me with these potentially contaminated onions.

To my playful accusation, she responded not with words but with laughter. I'd expected her to reassure me that the onions were perfectly safe, but instead, she just chuckled and walked away. Her enigmatic reaction momentarily left me pondering,

"Did I say something to upset her so much that she's willing to let me eat potentially toxic onions?"

Perplexed, I followed her into the family room, determined to get to the bottom of this lighthearted but mysterious onion ordeal. I asked, "Hun, you're really not trying to kill me, are you?" She responded with a sincere, "Of course not."

With a sigh of relief, I couldn't help but extend the jest. I asked her, "If you were trying to kill me, how would you do it?" She quickly retorted, "Onions, of course."

We both laughed at the weirdness of the situation, our worries dispelled by the playful banter. But then, a nagging thought crossed my mind. If these onions were so dangerous that they might actually kill me, then why wasn't my wife worried, given that she had eaten the same meal?

As we contemplated this conundrum, my wife delivered the final punchline. She simply said, "I didn't eat as many onions as you did, fatty." Her response sent us both into fits of laughter. It was a classic moment of marital humor that we would recall for years to come. These seemingly harmless onions would unwittingly set the stage for a profound turning point in my life, revealing the unexpected intricacies of my deteriorating health.

My story proceeds against the backdrop of a joyful family gathering at my brother's house. Laughter filled the air as the children played, and meaningful conversations flowed. Beers were shared, marking the end of an era and celebrating the simple pleasures of life. It was a day filled with happiness and camaraderie.

Yet, as we raised our glasses to toast, little did I know that my health was about to take a sharp and unexpected nosedive. Unbeknownst to me, those onions, which had once been the subject of playful banter with my wife, would soon become a haunting symbol of my mysterious illness. That night awaking with cramping abdominal pains, rushing to bathroom with diarrhea, only to be stunned as I looked down at a toilet bowl filed with blood. For I am about to face one of the most challenging and perplexing times of my life.

Chapter 3: The Torture Continues - Welcome to the Gates of Hell

As my body continued its relentless descent into the abyss of torment, I found myself trapped in a never-ending nightmare. Chronic diarrhea, abdominal discomfort, and bewildering symptoms tormented my every waking moment. I was well past the point of desperation and longing for answers. At this stage, the pain and suffering had become unbearable, and I couldn't endure it any longer. The unending misery was taking its toll on me, both physically and mentally.

Amidst the COVID-19 pandemic that had already disrupted lives across the globe, I embarked on a journey into the world of healthcare, seeking relief from my affliction. It was a time when healthcare systems and hospitals were overwhelmed, but I couldn't postpone seeking help any longer. My very survival depended on finding answers and solutions to my mysterious ailment. Dehydration was creeping in, causing my vital signs to fluctuate dangerously.

In a small room at a walk-in clinic, I was greeted by a concerned physician assistant. Two weeks of suffering and recurring episodes of debilitating diarrhea were the undeniable proof of my plight. I was experiencing severe dehydration with a lost of 15 pounds, and elevated resting heart rate of 120 beats per minute. The walls of my world were closing in on me, and I was desperately clinging to any glimmer of hope that came my way.

I began to recount my harrowing journey, describing the relentless agony and discomfort I had experienced. The physician assistant listened attentively, realizing the gravity of the situation. It was clear that the time for action had come. We couldn't afford any more delays or uncertainties; my life was hanging by a thread.

After a thorough examination and a series of tests, the physician assistant reached a conclusion. A grave look crossed their face as they gently shared their concerns and suspicions. It was likely a gastrointestinal disorder, but the exact nature of it remained an enigma. To move forward, I needed to consult a specialist—a gastrointestinal expert who could untangle the web of symptoms that had ensnared my life.

The physician assistant acted swiftly, ordering an array of tests and investigations that would serve as a starting point for the impending consultations. Hope for relief, albeit faint, flickered within me as I left the clinic. The prospect of answers, of finding my way out of this living nightmare, gave me a renewed sense of purpose.

Days turned into nights, and my symptoms only grew more relentless. The walls of my home began to feel like prison bars, closing in around me as I was held captive by my own gastrointestinal emergencies. Breathing became a struggle, and the fear of what lay ahead was suffocating. My body was a battlefield, and it was losing the war.

As my condition deteriorated further, I found myself at a crossroads. With dehydration looming over me and my vital signs indicating a crisis, I decided to heed the advice I had received and seek out the expertise of a gastrointestinal specialist.

The journey to the emergency room was a treacherous path to navigate, especially amid the chaos of a world gripped by the pandemic. As I sat in the waiting room, I couldn't help but wonder how many others were sharing this same journey, seeking solace from their torment, and grappling with uncertainty.

Finally, my name was called, and I was ushered into the examination room. I shared my unrelenting suffering with the doctor, emphasizing the urgency of my situation and the need for immediate intervention. My persistence, however, was met with skepticism and an unsettling indifference. It was as though I was speaking to an empty void, and my pleas for help were falling on deaf ears.

As the minutes ticked by, I underwent a series of uncomfortable tests, including an EKG, digital rectum exam, needles to draw blood and IVs placement that left me feeling more vulnerable than ever. The anguish of my physical symptoms was compounded by the emotional pain of not being taken seriously. I couldn't shake the feeling that I was on the brink of a precipice, and no one else could truly understand the depth of my suffering.

In the emergency room, I found myself waging a battle not just against my ailment but against the cold, indifferent currents of a healthcare system stretched thin by the relentless waves of a global pandemic. Advocating for my own well-being was an uphill struggle, but I knew that giving in to despair was not an option.

This chapter is a snapshot of a pivotal moment in my journey, a time when the darkness of uncertainty loomed large. It serves as a testament to the courage and tenacity required when faced with a medical mystery. I was admitted to the hospital diagnosed with tachycardia and dehydration, the emergency room doctor admitted me to the hospital for IV fluids and a further evaluation. Little did I know that my quest for answers was far from over and that I would continue to encounter unforeseen challenges along this arduous path toward healing.

Chapter 4: Some of the Nicest People

I n the midst of this bewildering labyrinth called the healthcare system, I had the extraordinary privilege of encountering some of the most compassionate and empathetic individuals who would later become my guiding stars during this tumultuous medical odyssey. Their warmth, dedication, and unwavering support provided a flicker of hope in the dark abyss of my deteriorating health.

My journey towards healing found its genesis in a small, private room within the hospital—a modest oasis of comfort amidst the vast, unforgiving desert of my suffering. These walls, bearing silent witness to countless tales of pain and perseverance, seemed to resonate with the echoes of hope. It was in this room that I embarked on a journey of a thousand tests and examinations, each one carrying me closer to the elusive truth behind my ailment. Even the less-than-glamorous requests for stool specimens became slightly less humiliating thanks to the patience and empathy of the medical staff who administered them. They comprehended not only the physical but also the emotional turmoil I endured.

One particular doctor, an internal medicine specialist, appeared like a beacon of hope in the storm of uncertainty. As he walked into my room, he carried with him an aura of both confidence and empathy. Every word he spoke became a lifeline, and I clung to them as he unveiled the path to recovery. His calm and reassuring demeanor instilled in me a trust that had been sorely absent in my previous interactions with the healthcare system. In that pivotal moment, I dared to believe that maybe, just maybe, there was a way out of this labyrinth of suffering. The doctor assured me that a consultation with a gastrointestinal specialist was already underway, a glimmer of hope reignited within my heart.

However, the array of compassionate characters in my medical journey didn't conclude with that singular doctor. Throughout my hospital stay, I was repeatedly struck by the profound empathy and dedication of the medical team that enveloped me. Among them, a young internal medicine resident shone as a shining example of a future physician, marked by not only knowledge but also genuine empathy. The medical staff took the time to listen, truly listen, to my experiences and fears. Their capacity to connect with me on a human level, in the sterile and busy inpatient hospital setting, proved to be invaluable during those turbulent times.

Before the colonoscopy and endoscopy, there were preparations to be undertaken, and the hospital staff kindly introduced me to the infamous "Golytely" prep. This less-than-appetizing solution, a necessary evil, was the final step in ensuring my readiness for the forthcoming procedures. The process was arduous, but I recognized it as a small price to pay for the potential answers that awaited me.

In the hospital room on the night before the invasive examinations, a tidal wave of gratitude overwhelmed me. The long hours of discomfort, uncertainty, and pain were about to be subjected to the ultimate litmus test—literally. The mere promise of a full night's rest, a luxury I had been denied for so long, was akin to a soothing balm for my anxious soul.

This chapter draws to a close as I find myself being wheeled towards the endoscopy/colonoscopy department, my mind a swirling vortex of emotions—anxiety intertwined with a resolute determination. The medication administered to quell my racing heart and restless thoughts proved insufficient. But in the midst of this turbulent sea, I was surrounded by the kind faces of the hospital staff. Their warm smiles and reassuring words provided me with the strength to carry on. In that moment, the path ahead appeared challenging, yes, but strangely manageable. The individuals I had encountered during my journey had the remarkable ability to transform what could have been an overwhelming experience into something I could endure.

Chapter 5: Last Few Days in the Hospital

A wave of relief washed over me after my first dose of IV steroids, solumedrol, coursed through my veins. It marked the beginning of my four-day stay in the hospital, where I transitioned from IV steroids to oral prednisone. It was during these pivotal days that the winds of change finally blew in my favor. I could feel my body responding positively to the treatment. My bowel movements became less of an incessant, unpredictable storm, and the cramping, bloating, and pain that had relentlessly tormented me began to subside. The path to recovery was becoming more discernible, and the horizon seemed brighter.

What made this stretch in the hospital more bearable were the remarkable nurses who graced my journey with their delightful presence. In the solemn and often somber hospital environment, their humor acted as a beacon of light, providing moments of respite from the ceaseless grind of medical procedures and treatments. Together, we shared genuine laughter, a healing elixir for the soul. These moments were as therapeutic as any medication, if not more so. And it was during this time that I found myself, at times, walking up and down the hallway in an open-back patient gown, sipping yellow Gatorade from a rather unconventional container—urinal. The weirdness of the situation never failed to spark a chuckle, turning what could have been an embarrassing moment into a cherished memory.

But it was more than humor that made those days in the hospital memorable. It was the genuine connections I formed with the medical staff who tended to my needs. One individual stood out among the healthcare heroes—the GI Doctor. His unwavering dedication to understanding my condition, especially my "shitty pics," as I referred to the photographic evidence of my struggles, was remarkable. It became a personal challenge, a source of amusement, to see how many people I could persuade to view my "poo gallery." I must say; the GI doctor was the most enthusiastic and empathetic viewer, proving that even in the realm of medicine, a bit of humor and camaraderie can work wonders.

As the days unfolded and my condition showed signs of improvement, I eagerly shared positive updates with the medical team. Each step forward was a glimmer of hope, a ray of sunshine breaking through the storm clouds. With fewer daily bowel movements, an overall sense of well-being, and an improving appetite, it seemed like I was on an upward trajectory. However, the certainty of my diagnosis remained elusive.

The biopsy results hinted at ulcerative colitis, but a conclusive diagnosis demanded more in-depth examination and investigation. The situation grew more complex as the colonoscopy had to be stopped due to excessive swelling and fragility of walls of my bowels, making it impossible to navigate through my sigmoid colon. This limitation meant that the rest of my colon could not be examined, adding difficulty to the diagnostic process.

With an insatiable thirst for knowledge and a commitment

to taking an active role in my health, I dived headfirst into researching inflammatory bowel disease, with a specific focus on ulcerative colitis. The internet became my ally and adversary, offering a trove of conflicting information. This digital exploration was a pivotal moment in my journey. It was a realization that my health was ultimately in my hands. It wasn't about following my doctor's guidance blindly; it was about forging a partnership with my healthcare providers, engaging in open dialogues about my health, and, most importantly, advocating for my well-being. I had long learned that it was not just acceptable but essential to challenge your doctor when the situation demanded it. And so, my quest for understanding and empowerment continued as I ventured further into the intricate and often perplexing world of inflammatory bowel disease.

Chapter 6: How to Improve Your Condition

I'm excited to share with you the invaluable strategies I've uncovered during my journey. These insights are not the product of medical wisdom but carry the weight of personal experience. It's the wisdom that's borne out of enduring suffering and ultimately emerging on the other side stronger and wiser. These strategies are not limited to managing inflammatory bowel disease but applicable to a healthy lifestyle in general.

The journey towards a brighter health future begins with a transformation of the mind—a shift in perspective that recognizes the immense power of positivity in the face of life's formidable challenges. It's about adopting a "can-do" attitude, understanding that many of life's stressors simply aren't worth the excessive worry they often trigger.

Stress is not just a mental battle; it has profound physiological effects. One of its most insidious impacts is the release of the stress hormone cortisol. A key pillar in managing and improving your condition is learning to lower your cortisol levels. One powerful way to achieve this is by prioritizing sleep. Think of sleep as the body's reset button—a time when it repairs, rejuvenates, and readies itself for the challenges of a new day.

Sleep's restorative effects can't be overstated. While the National Sleep Foundation offers specific recommendations for sleep durations based on age, a consistent aim for 7-9 hours of sleep per night is a reliable rule of thumb for most adults. That's your foundation for well-being, a time when your body repairs, your immune system strengthens, and your mind unwinds.

Challenging self-defeating thoughts is another critical aspect of improving your condition. It's about self-reflection, recognizing these negative thoughts when they arise, evaluating their accuracy, and then working on changing your perspective. Instead of an aggressive mindset, strive to be assertive. An assertive approach aids in effective communication, ensuring your needs are met while respecting the needs of others.

Physical activity, too, plays a vital role in maintaining your physical and emotional health. It's about incorporating a balanced amount of exercise into your daily routine. This includes a combination of moderate aerobic exercise and resistance training. For those who are ready to push their limits, high-intensity interval training (HIIT) can be an efficient choice. Exercise isn't just about fitness; it's about the release of endorphins, those magical neurotransmitters that make you feel good and help battle the blues.

The importance of stress management techniques can't be emphasized enough in your quest for well-being. Relaxation is a powerful tool to keep stress at bay. This involves embracing mindful meditation, deep breathing exercises, and activities that help you unwind and find calmness. But remember, it's not just about managing stress; it's about finding joy and laughter in your life. It's about exploring new hobbies, embracing your passions, and taking the time for things that make you truly happy.

Another fundamental pillar of well-being is maintaining healthy relationships. It involves open and honest communication, trust, and the ability to navigate conflicts successfully. Being reliable, responsible, and respecting the needs and boundaries of both yourself and others is a part of this complex equation.

The path to personal growth and wellness involves multifaceted steps. It's about learning from your failures, embracing self-improvement, and recognizing the significance of personal development. On this journey, spirituality plays a vital role. Whether it's through prayer, meditation, or simple acts of kindness, spirituality helps you maintain a connection to something greater, a force that can offer solace and strength as you navigate the twists and turns of life.

Lastly, in this chapter, I introduce a topic that we'll delve into more deeply in a subsequent chapter: the importance of a healthy diet. It's about adopting a holistic approach to improving your condition and taking charge of your health. The journey to better health is dynamic, multifaceted, and often filled with twists and turns. However, armed with these strategies and insights, you can chart a course towards improved health and a life well-lived.

Chapter 7: Going Home

The day had finally arrived when I received the much-anticipated approval for discharge from the hospital. It was a momentous step in my journey towards reclaiming my health and embracing a future filled with vitality and well-being.

The process of leaving the hospital, I discovered, is a meticulously orchestrated affair. Doctors' orders, instructions for post-hospital care, and a list of essential medications are sent to your designated pharmacy. To ensure a smooth transition, it's advisable to call your pharmacy ahead of time, verifying that all the necessary prescriptions have been transmitted electronically. In my case, this step turned out to be quite crucial, as it would save me the hassle of delays or misunderstandings when I was finally home.

As I prepared to embark on the ride back to my sanctuary, I was filled with a whirlwind of emotions. The overarching feeling was one of profound relief that my days in the hospital were drawing to a close. No longer would I be confined to sterile rooms, the constant hum of machines, or the scrutiny of an ever-watchful medical team. It was an opportunity to return to the comforting familiarity of my own space and regain a sense of autonomy that had been momentarily ceded to the hospital's care.

Yet, accompanying this relief was a sense of apprehension. My hospital stay had left a significant impact on my physical condition. The severe illness I had endured, coupled with a myriad of medications, had resulted in a noticeable loss of weight. My body, once familiar and predictable, felt altered and fragile. It was clear that my lifestyle needed a profound overhaul, and the choices I made in the days and weeks to come would be instrumental in the trajectory of my recovery.

The hospitalization had provided a respite from my usual routine. It had separated me from the poor dietary choices, the excessive consumption of coffee, and the patterns of physical inactivity that had, in part, led me to that hospital bed. Returning to the environment that had contributed to my condition was, in essence, returning to the scene of the crime. I couldn't continue down the same path if I hoped to achieve lasting recovery.

My father, a pillar of unwavering support throughout this arduous journey, arrived to pick me up from the hospital. The car ride back home became an opportunity for an open and heartfelt conversation, one that was laden with my fears, concerns, and a shared commitment to my well-being.

The importance of family support can never be overstated. My father's presence was a testament to the unshakable bond that exists within a family. He recognized that my return home marked the beginning of a new chapter in our lives. His understanding, love, and encouragement were vital as we discussed the challenges and changes that lay ahead.

The car trip was a pivotal moment in my journey towards recovery. It was a dialogue that brought clarity to my intentions. I shared my apprehensions about maintaining the changes needed to improve my health and expressed my fears of falling back into old habits. These open and honest discussions were a testament to the strength of family bonds and the shared commitment to a healthier future.

This was the inception of a new chapter in my life, one that I was determined to write with purpose and resilience. I had a newfound understanding of the importance of taking control of my health. The decisions I made from this point forward were not solely for my benefit but also for the well-being of those I held dear.

As we approached home, I knew that my voyage was far from over. It was merely transitioning to a different phase, one that involved daily choices and a steadfast commitment to a healthier way of living. My recovery would be an ongoing process, a testament to the resilience of the human spirit and the profound impact that determination, love, and support can have on one's life.

In the confines of my home, I could feel the weight of responsibility and possibility pressing upon me. It was the beginning of a chapter that I was determined to fill with stories of healing, strength, and the reclamation of a life worth living. My trek continued, but now it was a journey towards health, happiness, and a future of boundless potential.

Chapter 8: My Journey Through Dietary Challenges

I n the quiet of the hospital room, I had embarked on an exploration of knowledge, determined to uncover the keys to managing my condition. My days became filled with sifting through an ever-growing stack of low-FODMAP diet recipes. This peculiar regimen was a dietary strategy recommended to soothe the flames of inflammatory bowel disease. The acronym "FODMAP" stood for "Fermentable Oligo-, Di-, Mono-saccharides And Polyols." These were the elusive short-chain carbohydrates (sugars) that wreaked havoc on my intestines, eagerly absorbing water and fermenting in my colon.

Upon deeper research, it became apparent that this diet was primarily aimed at patients grappling with irritable bowel syndrome (IBS). Its promise was to reduce the uncomfortable digestive symptoms – bloating, flatulence, and abdominal discomfort. However, the list of forbidden foods seemed to stretch on indefinitely, with some familiar foes including onions, garlic, shallots, and a host of other items known to send my gut into disarray. Avoiding this dietary rogue's gallery was undeniably my best course of action.

Thus began my culinary odyssey, a journey that would take

me through a maze of dietary restrictions, and it was here that my exploration of food began. After a painful flare-up, I wholeheartedly embraced weeks of commitment to a low-FODMAP diet, carefully navigating each meal to avoid the dietary triggers that had wrought havoc on my body.

But this was not the end of my cooking adventures. No, I decided to combine the low-FODMAP diet with the delightful Mediterranean Diet, a culinary fusion that held the promise of delicious and nourishing meals. Not to contradict the Mediterranean diet, I did have to say farewell to nuts, seeds, and the notorious onions that had tormented me. In their place, I welcomed leeks as trusty substitute. It was an experiment that would ultimately bring me relief and a cooking experience that extended beyond my expectations.

Through these culinary experiments, I was able to transform what might have been seen as a limited diet into a journey of cuisine creativity. The restrictions were challenging, but they served as a catalyst for my culinary inventiveness.

One of the key lessons I learned during this time was the importance of consuming foods that were as close to their natural state as possible. Processed foods, laden with preservatives, were to be avoided. I realized that it was time for me to take charge of my diet, and that meant making food from scratch as often as possible. As it turned out, the age-old adage held true – "You are what you eat." Making my own meals allowed me to control the quality and freshness of the ingredients I consumed.

One aspect that I couldn't stress enough was the value of a vacuum food sealer. Preparing large meals was a staple in my kitchen. To ensure that nothing went to waste, I would freeze individual portions in vacuum-sealed bags. This not only preserved the flavor and quality of my dishes but also made meal planning incredibly convenient.

When it came to warming up my homemade creations, I had a clear favorite – the trusty toaster oven. It offered a unique advantage over the microwave; the food tasted better. There had always been a cloud of doubt regarding the impact of microwaves on food quality and health, and though the Food and Drug Administration's stance on microwave safety had eased some concerns, my loyalty firmly rested with the oven and stove.

However, life is often a whirlwind, and time is a precious commodity. In my quest for a balance between home-cooked meals and convenience, I stumbled upon the glorious world of meal delivery services. The market was brimming with options, and I meticulously combed through ingredient lists, ensuring that the food I consumed met my dietary requirements. Trifecta, with its focus on organic, non-GMO produce and pre-prepared meals, became a personal favorite. Modify Health was another notable contender, offering organic, non-GMO fare, alongside grass-fed and wild-caught proteins. Epicured delivery, with its gluten-free and additive-free offerings, also proved to be a star player in this culinary arena.

However, amidst all these convenient options, the most profound realization dawned on me – that the finest culinary adventure unfolds right in the heart of one's own kitchen. Initially, I had felt guilty about dedicating so much time to cooking. I worried that my son was missing out on quality time with me. But then, the perfect solution revealed itself – why not make cooking a joint activity?

This revelation transformed the way I approached my culinary endeavors. I invited my four-year-old son to be my little sous chef, and to my delight, he eagerly accepted the invitation. He reveled in measuring ingredients, pouring, and stirring. Our culinary escapades became bonding sessions, peppered with giggles and heartwarming conversations. The bonus? He began to devour vegetables he'd previously shunned, marking a small yet significant victory in our culinary journey.

As you explore the chapters ahead, you'll discover a treasure trove of recipes that won't demand hours of toil in the kitchen, the perfect complement to this culinary adventure of mine. The path to health, I learned, is also a journey of creative and satisfying meals that nourish the body and soul. It's a testament to the enduring connection between food, well-being, and the joy of sharing culinary experiences with those you love.

Chapter 9: A Painful Twist in the Tale

B ack at home after my hospital stay, I had hoped for a return to normalcy. Unfortunately, life had a different plan for me. A strange discomfort began to settle in, originating from my leg. It felt as though my veins were orchestrating a peculiar symphony of pain, with the saphenous vein in my calf taking center stage.

Naturally, I decided to pay a visit to my family practice doctor, eager to unravel this new mystery that had woven itself into my post-hospital life. My weight loss journey had brought along some unwelcome companions – varicose veins, where there had been none before. My doctor, noting my pain and the unusual hardness in my vein, decided it was time for some medical exploration. An ultrasound was ordered for my right leg, scheduled for the next morning.

Now, that ultrasound appointment was memorable, but not for the right reasons. As I lay there, a kind yet insistent technician began her work. She asked me to undress, and in my discomfort, I obliged. The procedure was, to say the least, excruciating, with compression techniques that nearly brought me to tears. But to my surprise, the spot where my pain resided remained untouched. When I inquired, she nonchalantly declared, "We are all done." I persisted, but she remained firm in her declaration.

The following day, my leg's torment escalated, the pain climbing up to my groin. It was a call to action. I rang my doctor, and he arranged another scan for Monday. The second ultrasound experience was equally bewildering, with a technician whose attitude bore hints of irritation. "Back so soon?" she quipped. Frustrated, I recounted my experiences and learned the shocking truth – they didn't scan superficial veins. Their protocol, it seemed, excluded these critical investigations.

But I couldn't accept this response. I argued that a clot could be life-threatening, and months of waiting for a vascular specialist wasn't an option. We locked horns, and she reluctantly began the scan, revealing a worrying presence of clots throughout my femoral vein. It's crucial to seek medical attention if you suspect a femoral vein clot or experience symptoms such as persistent leg swelling, pain, or warmth. Timely diagnosis and appropriate treatment can help prevent complications and reduce the risk of serious health issues associated with femoral vein clots.

Femoral vein clots, also known as deep vein thrombosis (DVT) in the femoral vein, can pose serious health risks. Here are some potential dangers associated with femoral vein clots:

1. **Pulmonary Embolism (PE):** One of the most severe complications of femoral vein clots is the risk of a pulmonary embolism. If a clot dislodges from the femoral vein and travels to the lungs, it can block blood flow, leading to a potentially life-threatening situation.
2. **Compromised Blood Flow:** A femoral vein clot can impede or block blood flow in the affected leg, causing pain, swelling, and potentially leading to chronic issues such as post-thrombotic syndrome.

3. **Chronic Venous Insufficiency:** Untreated femoral vein clots may result in chronic venous insufficiency, a condition where the valves in the veins are damaged, leading to long-term problems with blood circulation in the legs.
4. **Recurrence of Clots:** Individuals who have experienced a femoral vein clot may be at an increased risk of developing further clots in the future.
5. **Infection:** Clots can increase the risk of infection in the affected area, especially if the clot causes damage to the blood vessel wall.
6. **Leg Swelling and Pain:** Femoral vein clots can cause significant swelling and pain in the affected leg, impacting mobility and overall quality of life.

My faith was somewhat restored when a familiar face from my previous appointment wheeled me over to my doctor's office. The physician recognized the gravity of the situation, acknowledging the unacceptable negligence I had experienced. With empathy and apologies, he outlined a path forward. I was prescribed Xarelto, a blood thinner, and a follow-up appointment was scheduled in three weeks.

To add a touch of humor, I couldn't resist a light-hearted jab at my doctor about spending so much time together it may make your wife jealous. We both chuckled, lightening the mood amidst the tension. As we concluded the visit, I asked him to send my prescription to a pharmacy in the same building.

The journey didn't end there. I found myself at the pharmacy counter, where the nuances of insurance and prior authorization unveiled another layer of healthcare complexity. The process of getting my medication was fraught with bureaucracy and red tape. Despite the frustration, I was determined to navigate this maze and emerge on the other side with the treatment I needed.

During those three months on Xarelto, my life was filled with uncertainty. The pain in my leg was a constant reminder of the potential dangers lurking within my body. Every twinge and ache sent my mind racing with worry. The path to diagnosis and treatment was fraught with obstacles, and my health felt like a fragile house of cards.

As I left the hospital that day, I couldn't help but marvel at the resilience of the human spirit. Despite the challenges and frustrations, I was determined to regain my health and continue moving forward. My health had taken me on a journey I had never anticipated.

This chapter of my story serves as a reminder that the journey to health is rarely a straightforward path. It's filled with twists and turns, unexpected obstacles, and moments of frustration. Yet, it's also a testament to the strength of the human spirit and the importance of advocating for one's health. As I looked ahead to the next steps in my recovery, I knew that I would face them with determination and resilience, just as I had throughout my entire journey.

Chapter 10: An Unsettling Encounter With the Gastrointestinal Doctor

M eeting the GI (Gastrointestinal) doctor was a rather peculiar experience, to say the least. My appointment began with the nurse, who fired off a barrage of questions, took my vital signs, and recorded my weight. I had reached 165 pounds, a welcome gain from my lowest point at 147 pounds. But then came the doctor, and he turned out to be a walking contradiction – remarkably knowledgeable but disorganized to the point of chaos. It seemed like every time he had an idea, he would either summon his nurse or disappear from the room to call her, scribbling prescriptions haphazardly. The disarray left me feeling uneasy; it was a recipe for mistakes.

My first question was about my next colonoscopy. The doctor's response, "6 months to a year from now," didn't sit right with me. When I left the hospital, they suspected I had ulcerative colitis, but the pathology reports were inconclusive. Furthermore, my rectum appeared healthy, which was unusual for ulcerative colitis. I pressed him on this point, suspecting that there was more to my diagnosis than met the eye.

His solution to this uncertainty was an aggressive treatment plan involving methotrexate and Remicade infusion. In my mind, it felt like he was throwing the entire medical library at me. Methotrexate, typically used for cancer, arthritis, and psoriasis, was intended to suppress my immune system and stop it from attacking itself. The list of potential side effects read like a catalog of horrors, and I couldn't help but feel a growing sense of unease.

The second component of the treatment plan, Remicade, was an immune-suppressing biological drug targeting inflammation. While it had been approved in 2005, its side effects were no less daunting than methotrexate, including the risk of life-threatening infections and even cancer. What made this doubly concerning was the fact that once you start these medications, your body tends to form antibodies that prevent them from working as effectively if you ever stop. It felt like my treatment plan was on a one-way track, and my body might revolt in response.

I raised my concerns with the doctor, explaining my fears about such a potent treatment plan. As a father with young children and a career in the ICU working with seriously ill patients, the risks seemed immense. Additionally, I had received a positive Quantiferon test result indicating exposure to tuberculosis, which added another layer of concern. A suppressed immune system, especially in the midst of a tuberculosis scare, could spell disaster. My question was simple: were there any alternatives? I was looking for reassurance, some hope that there might be a less aggressive route.

The doctor's answer, however, was swift and final – this aggressive treatment was my best chance, and he provided no alternatives. I was left feeling like I was standing at a dead end with no other paths to explore. It was a moment of deep frustration and uncertainty.

Our conversation then took a turn as we discussed my colonoscopy images. I had seen them, and I knew that the situation was dire, but I also knew that we lacked a definitive diagnosis beyond the Sigmoid colon biopsy. Could this be diverticulitis, or environmental factors I wondered, or perhaps a severe food allergy? The doctor, however, deemed these possibilities highly unlikely. It was as though we were stuck in a labyrinth, with the doctor urging me to take a specific path while I was struggling to see the full landscape.

The doctor's suggestion to meet with a nutritionist was met with agreement, though I had to check if my insurance would cover such a consultation. We wrapped up the appointment, prescriptions were written, and I was scheduled for Remicade and Methotrexate. However, it would be some time before insurance would cover the infusions. The medication list included folic acid, zofran, and vitamin D, alongside the requirement for regular lab work every two weeks. The gravity of these decisions pressed heavily on me as I departed from the doctor's office.

This unsettling encounter with the gastrointestinal doctor had left me with a multitude of questions and a sense of disquiet. The treatment plan that had been laid out before me was formidable and came with its own set of potential perils. As I walked away from the appointment, I couldn't help but wonder if there might be other paths to explore, or if I was truly at the mercy of this one, despite the storm of uncertainties swirling around it.

Chapter 11: Regaining Control Over my Life

Returning home after the ordeal in the hospital, I was confronted with a pivotal decision. I realized that it was my body, my life, and I needed to be the one to take control of it. The changes I had initiated in Chapter 6, revolving around diet and lifestyle, had marked the beginning of a transformative journey.

As I gazed at my reflection in the mirror, I saw an emaciated, frail figure looking back at me – a stark contrast to the healthy, vigorous individual I had once been. The muscles I had painstakingly built were gone, replaced by the gauntness brought about by my illness. It was a sobering moment, but instead of succumbing to self-pity, I knew it was time for a fundamental shift in my perspective. The past few months could not define me. I needed to start anew, to rebuild not only my physical strength but my emotional resilience. It was no longer just about me; it was about being better for my wife and children. This disease, no matter how relentless, would not define my life.

In that moment, I found a deep well of determination within myself. I realized that I was in control, and I could choose to be more optimistic. My colon may have been damaged, but it was not beyond repair. The battle to heal had commenced, and I was going to be an active participant in it.

However, before I could fully commit to this path of healing, there was a lingering issue that needed resolution – my ongoing concerns regarding the GI doctor's treatment plan. I sent him a message, inquiring about any potential alternative treatments. My apprehensions about the side effects of Remicade and Methotrexate, the risks associated with immunosuppression, and the possibility of developing antibodies if I ever needed to stop the treatment were all genuine concerns. My substantial lifestyle changes had been having a positive impact, and I was beginning to feel better. Additionally, I questioned the possibility of severe food allergies, environmental factors or diverticulitis, which could be valid explanations for my condition. The response I received from the doctor's nurse did little to alleviate my concerns – I was informed that the medications were the only way to prevent the need for surgery. But I couldn't simply accept that as the final verdict.

Determined to explore all my options, I made a call to the doctor's office, requesting a direct conversation with him. The secretary conveyed that he was occupied but assured me that he would call me back. Hours passed with an air of uncertainty before my phone rang, and it was the doctor on the line. I laid out my apprehensions regarding Remicade and Methotrexate, emphasizing my concerns about potential side effects and the looming specter of immunosuppression. I explained my fears for my children, my own exposure to tuberculosis, my age, and the side effects of these medications. I stressed the point that the absence of any imaging showing improvement was troubling. My persistence paid off, and the doctor ultimately ordered an MRI Enterography (MRE) to obtain a clearer view of my intestines.

Despite this glimmer of hope, it was evident that I needed more than just an additional diagnostic test. I needed a fresh perspective, a second opinion. The doctor had been resolute in his prescription of Remicade and Methotrexate, but I couldn't shake the feeling that there had to be another way. Our interactions had left me feeling dismissed and disheartened, and that led me to conclude that seeking another healthcare professional's input was the next logical step on my journey to recovery. This thought became the guiding light, steering me toward an alternative path, one that was hopeful and promising, despite the challenges that lay ahead.

Chapter 12: The MRI

O n the day of my scheduled MRI, I was filled with a mixture of anticipation and nervousness. It was an early start, and I made my way to the hospital, only to find myself in the waiting room once again. It's quite ironic how one rushes to a place only to spend a significant amount of time waiting. While in the waiting area, I decided to make productive use of this unexpected idle time by working on another chapter for this book.

After a considerable wait, they called my name, and I was ushered in for the MRI procedure. The medical staff explained the process, and I was then directed to secure my personal belongings in a locker. From there, I was led into the IV room for placement.

Next on the agenda was the consumption of oral contrast, a type of contrast agent used in gastrointestinal evaluations. Due to legal reasons, I won't mention its name, but I can confidently say it's something I would prefer not to ingest again. The list of ingredients included a variety of questionable substances and additives that were in stark contrast to the fresh unprocessed healthy diet that I have embraced. It was an unappetizing concoction, to say the least. I found myself pondering whether consuming this oral contrast was any less appealing than some other gastrointestinal evaluation methods.

The aftermath of this unappetizing experience was a different story. Within a mere 45 minutes, my stomach began to protest with discomfort, cramps, and a general sense of malaise. These sensations persisted for the next two hours, making the MRI experience that much more challenging and unpleasant. Yet, my focus remained on the medical procedures and the goal of finding answers to my health concerns. These unexpected moments, my journey was still unfolding, and I had more to discover and conquer. The MRI was just another chapter in the larger narrative of my quest for answers and healing.

Chapter 13: Virtual Visits and the GI Doctor

My journey through the healthcare system had taken an unexpected turn as my GI doctor decided to transition to virtual visits. In the age of digital connectivity, virtual appointments have become increasingly common, providing convenience and flexibility for both doctors and patients. However, my experience with this particular virtual visit would prove to be far from routine.

I found myself seated in front of my computer, the anticipation of a critical discussion with my GI doctor building as each minute passed. The doctor, despite being a staggering 50 minutes late to our scheduled appointment, finally appeared on my screen. Now, being kept waiting by doctors is somewhat of a common quirk in the healthcare world, but what unfolded during this virtual visit was far from the usual.

To begin, I felt it was only polite to inquire about the doctor's well-being, expecting a courteous response. However, his reply was curt and dismissive, setting the tone for the rest of our interaction. I proceeded to discuss the results of my MRI and shared my experiences of improved health with only one bowel movement a day. To my surprise, his response was far from what I had hoped for. "You already read the report," he stated.

While the hospital had provided online access to the reports, merely reading them didn't imply that I fully comprehended their significance. I had questions, genuine concerns that I needed him to address. But instead of providing clarity, he offered only vague answers, leaving me in a state of confusion and frustration.

When I asked if there was any improvement based on the MRI results, his response was nothing short of disheartening. He declared my condition as severe and bluntly stated that my options were limited to taking biological medications or undergoing surgery. I was utterly taken aback by this prognosis, considering the significant turnaround I had experienced and what I had read in the radiologist's report. It was as though the doctor's conclusion was predetermined, without any consideration for the progress I had made.

The virtual visit left me deeply unsettled, and I couldn't shake the feeling that something was off. It was time to get that second opinion, a fresh perspective to navigate my way through this complex medical landscape. I had already received a recommendation from a close family friend who had been battling inflammatory bowel disease for over a decade. This friend had endured a long and challenging journey, and his experience was invaluable. I was determined to explore my options beyond the narrow path laid out by my current doctor.

During the virtual visit, I had also requested specific lab work to be done, which was essential for my condition. This included tests for vitamin D, iron, comprehensive metabolic panel (CMP), various B vitamins, folate, and C-reactive protein (CRP). The intention was to have a comprehensive understanding of my overall health, tailored to my situation. Initially, the doctor displayed reluctance, but eventually, he wrote the necessary orders for the requested lab work.

Another point of concern was the absence of a baseline esophagogastroduodenoscopy (EGD) or a colonoscopy. Instead, he proposed a sigmoidoscopy, which fell short of what I believed was required for a thorough evaluation. It was becoming increasingly clear that we weren't on the same page when it came to the approach and the level of scrutiny necessary for my diagnosis.

Our conversation delved into the treatment plan. When the doctor inquired if I would be willing to take medication, my response was negative. I explained my intention to explore alternative/functional medicine and consider allergist options. Alternative medicine, in my view, focused on optimizing the body's functioning and the health of its organs, which I believed was a valid and valuable approach.

However, my doctor's response was far from receptive. He appeared visibly annoyed and, in a hurried manner, declared that he had to go, terminating our conversation abruptly. I thanked him, although it was likely that he recognized the sarcasm in my tone. This virtual visit marked the end of our professional relationship. I knew I was moving forward to explore new horizons in my quest for answers and healing. This doctor's aggressive approach raised concerns, as it could potentially be harmful unless I was willing to think outside the box and take control of my health. The virtual visit left me with more questions than answers, but it also ignited a fire within me to seek out a doctor who could provide the care and understanding that I deserved.

Chapter 14: Gathering Allies and Embracing Herbal Wisdom

I n the early stages of my health journey, I grappled with the reluctance to discuss my health issues with those close to me. The embarrassment associated with my condition was a significant hurdle I had to overcome. As I began to open up, however, I discovered the wealth of knowledge and support that awaited me from friends, family, and acquaintances. Many of them were eager to help and offered their insights, some of whom had personal experience dealing with inflammatory bowel disease. These conversations transformed my perspective and provided me with valuable advice and even recommendations.

One particular conversation stands out in my memory. I spoke with a close friend who had been battling Crohn's disease for over a decade, enduring numerous bowel resections and medical interventions. I decided to give him an abridged version of my health journey, feeling somewhat vulnerable about discussing the details. To my surprise, he was not only empathetic but also incredibly informative. He provided me with invaluable suggestions, shared stories of his own struggles, and even introduced me to a trusted GI doctor. This introduction came as a ray of hope, and without hesitation, I made an appointment with this new doctor, mentally preparing myself for what I believed would be another treatment plan akin to the one from the difficult GI doctor.

The day of the appointment with the new GI doctor arrived, and I embarked on the 40-minute drive to his clinic. This time, I resolved to let him take the lead in our conversation, answer his questions comprehensively, and provide all the subjective data I could. I walked into the clinic with positive expectations, fueled by the glowing recommendations I had received. The atmosphere in the waiting room seemed different from my previous experiences, exuding professionalism and a sense of reliability.

When the GI doctor finally entered the patient's room, I greeted him with enthusiasm. I conveyed my eagerness to have him as my GI doctor, based on the positive feedback I had received and my desire to move forward with confidence in my treatment. He greeted me with a warm smile and immediately began asking questions, demonstrating a genuine interest in my well-being. He carefully reviewed my detailed medical history, taking note of the fact that I was not taking Remicade, the biological drug that had been prescribed by the previous GI doctor. His expression mirrored my confusion about why such a potent medication had been recommended, especially when it appeared that I was experiencing a period of remission, as I had described. The new doctor concurred with my sentiments and assured me that while the medication might be considered in the future, it was not necessary at this moment.

Our conversation continued, with the GI doctor meticulously explaining that I should continue with my current medication regimen of Colazal (Balsalazide) since I was doing well on it. He emphasized that I could reach out to him if I encountered any issues, and he shared his impressive track record of keeping 90% of his patients out of the hospital. This was music to my ears, reinforcing my optimism about the potential partnership.

We engaged in an in-depth discussion about the results of my CT and MRI scans, with the doctor providing detailed insights into the findings. I couldn't help but ask if there was a noticeable improvement between the CT scan and the MRI or magnetic resonance enterography (MRE). His response was affirming – there was indeed improvement, although inflammation still persisted. This news was a relief, offering concrete evidence that my journey towards recovery was on the right track.

During our appointment, I also raised my concern about the absence of a baseline esophagogastroduodenoscopy (EGD) or a full colonoscopy, essential procedures for a comprehensive evaluation of my condition. The doctor readily acknowledged this oversight and assured me that we would arrange for these procedures in the coming month. This was an essential step in establishing a thorough understanding of my gastrointestinal health and ensuring that no potential issues went unnoticed.

The topic of probiotics also came up during our conversation, and I was delighted to find that the GI doctor not only supported their use but also provided specific recommendations. He enthusiastically endorsed the use of probiotics, specifically recommending two brands: VSL#3 and Visbiome. This recommendation emphasized the doctor's commitment to exploring holistic and natural approaches to managing my condition.

As I left the clinic that day, my heart was filled with a newfound sense of optimism. This appointment marked the beginning of a fresh chapter in my battle against the disease, and I felt prepared to face the challenges ahead. It was reassuring to realize that my evolving understanding of my condition and its management was aligning with the perspectives of this new GI doctor. The importance of gathering allies and embracing herbal wisdom had become evident on my path to recovery, and I was ready to navigate the complexities of this journey with renewed hope and confidence.

Chapter 15: Embracing Alternative Medicine and the Herbal Heroes

B efore we delve into this somewhat contentious chapter, it's crucial to make a few important disclaimers. First and foremost, I am not a medical doctor, and the content of this book is by no means a substitute for professional medical advice. My intention is solely to share my personal journey, offering insight into the positive progress I made by embracing an alternative medicine approach. It is essential to recognize that what works for one individual may not work for another, and any significant changes in healthcare should always be done under the guidance of a healthcare professional.

Alternative medicine goes by various names, such as functional medicine, complementary medicine, or integrative medicine. It differs from conventional medicine in that it doesn't just aim to manage symptoms but seeks to understand the root causes of illnesses. This approach delves into the "how" and "why" behind symptoms and looks into the origins of diseases. In essence, alternative medicine adopts a holistic perspective on health, addressing not only the physical aspects but also mental, emotional, social, spiritual, and environmental factors that impact overall well-being.

Exploring Herbal Wisdom

One cornerstone of alternative medicine that I embarked upon was the realm of herbal remedies. Nature, with its vast array of plants and herbs, has been a source of healing for centuries. Different cultures across the globe have harnessed the therapeutic properties of various plants to treat and prevent ailments. This age-old knowledge has been passed down through generations, creating a treasury of herbal wisdom.

The Power of Herbal Medicine

Herbal medicine revolves around the use of plants, plant extracts, and plant-based substances to promote health and well-being. The origins of herbal medicine can be traced back to ancient civilizations in Egypt, China, India, and Greece, where healers relied heavily on the medicinal properties of plants.

As my journey to better health continued, I decided to explore the possibilities offered by herbal remedies. I was drawn to the idea of tapping into nature's own pharmacy, seeking potential allies in the plant kingdom to complement my treatment regimen. Here are some of the herbal heroes that played a significant role in my journey:

- Aloe Vera: Aloe vera is renowned for its soothing properties, particularly for gastrointestinal issues. It can reduce inflammation in the digestive tract and alleviate symptoms of inflammatory bowel disease. I started incorporating aloe vera juice into my daily routine, experiencing its calming effects on my gut.
- Turmeric: The active compound in turmeric, curcumin, is a potent anti-inflammatory agent. It has been extensively studied for its potential benefits in inflammatory bowel

48

diseases. I began adding turmeric to my meals and occasionally took curcumin supplements under the guidance of my healthcare providers.

- Slippery Elm: Slippery elm, with its mucilaginous properties, can provide relief for a sore and inflamed gastrointestinal tract. It forms a soothing gel when mixed with water and consumed. This natural remedy offered me comfort during flare-ups.
- Chamomile: Chamomile is renowned for its calming and contributed to a noticeable reduction in inflammation. It can help alleviate digestive discomfort and reduce stress, which can be a trigger for inflammatory bowel diseases. I enjoyed chamomile tea as part of my daily routine.
- Boswellia: Boswellia, also known as Indian frankincense, has anti-inflammatory properties and may support gut health. It's commonly used in Ayurvedic medicine for its potential benefits in managing inflammatory conditions.
- Licorice Root: Licorice root can help soothe the gastrointestinal lining and reduce inflammation. Do not use it if one has high blood pressure. Only for short term use.
- Marshmallow Root: Similar to slippery elm, marshmallow root's mucilaginous properties provide relief for a sore and inflamed gut. It can help protect the gastrointestinal lining.
- Probiotic- Visobiome can help alleviate various digestive issues, such as constipation, bloating, and gas. They are also used in the treatment of certain gastrointestinal conditions like inflammatory bowel disease (IBD).

The Role of Herbal Medicine in My Healing Journey

The integration of herbal remedies into my daily routine was a gradual process, and I always ensured that I consulted with healthcare providers before making any significant changes. These herbal allies were not meant to replace conventional medications but to complement them, enhancing my overall well-being.

As I incorporated these herbal heroes into my regimen, I observed several positive changes:

- Reduced Inflammation: Many of the herbs I used, such as turmeric, aloe vera, and chamomile, have anti-inflammatory properties. They contributed to a noticeable reduction in inflammation, particularly in my gut.
- Digestive Comfort: Herbs like slippery elm and marshmallow root offered soothing relief during flare-ups, helping ease discomfort and pain associated with my condition.
- Stress Management: Chamomile, with its calming properties, played a crucial role in managing stress, a common trigger for inflammatory bowel diseases.
- Support for Medications: Some herbal remedies worked in harmony with my prescribed medications to alleviate symptoms and improve overall digestive health.
- Enhanced Well-Being: By embracing herbal wisdom, I experienced a sense of empowerment in managing my health. It allowed me to take an active role in my healing journey.

Finding Balance

While herbal remedies provide significant benefits, it's essential to emphasize that the integration of these natural allies should be a collaborative decision with healthcare providers. Herbal supplements can interact with medications and have varying effects on individuals. Therefore, a healthcare provider's guidance is invaluable in ensuring the safe and effective use of herbal medicine.

Moreover, it's crucial to remember that herbal medicine is not a one-size-fits-all solution. What works for one person may not work for another. Our bodies and health conditions are unique, and the approach to herbal remedies should be tailored accordingly.

The Power of Nutrition

Another fundamental aspect of my alternative medicine journey was a focus on nutrition. As I delved deeper into the principles of functional medicine, I recognized the pivotal role that food plays in our health. The food we consume acts as fuel for our bodies, impacting our overall well-being, and can significantly influence the management of inflammatory bowel diseases.

The Impact of Diet on Inflammatory Bowel Diseases

Inflammatory bowel diseases, such as Crohn's disease and ulcerative colitis, are complex conditions with various triggers and factors that can exacerbate symptoms. While diet alone may not be a cure, it can play a significant role in symptom management and overall health.

A diet tailored to the needs of individuals with inflammatory bowel diseases should consider the following factors:

- Inflammation: Certain foods can trigger or exacerbate inflammation in the gastrointestinal tract. An anti-inflammatory diet can help reduce inflammation and relieve symptoms.
- Nutrient Absorption: Inflammatory bowel diseases can

hinder the absorption of essential nutrients. Therefore, a diet that ensures optimal nutrient absorption is crucial for overall health.

- Fiber Content: The choice of dietary fiber can significantly impact digestive health. High-fiber foods can be beneficial for some individuals, but they may exacerbate symptoms in others.

- FODMAPs: Some people with inflammatory bowel diseases are sensitive to FODMAPs (fermentable oligosaccharides, disaccharides, monosaccharides, and polyols), which are certain types of carbohydrates found in various foods. Reducing FODMAP intake can help manage symptoms.

- Trigger Foods: Different individuals may have specific trigger foods that worsen their symptoms. Identifying and avoiding these trigger foods is an essential aspect of dietary management.

- Hydration: Staying well-hydrated is crucial, especially for individuals with diarrhea, as they may lose excess fluids. Proper hydration can help maintain digestive health.

- Balanced Nutrition: A balanced diet that provides all essential nutrients is vital for overall health. It should include proteins, healthy fats, (healthy) carbohydrates, vitamins, and minerals.

By considering these factors, individuals with inflammatory bowel diseases can make informed dietary choices to help manage their condition and improve their quality of life. Please consult with a healthcare provider or registered dietitian for personalized dietary recommendations based on your specific condition and needs.

Chapter 16: The Healing Power of Food - A Journey to Wellness

I n my quest for better health, I unearthed a trove of wisdom that transcended traditional medical approaches. The nurse practitioner from functional medicine that I encountered became my guiding light, leading me toward a path less traveled but filled with promise.

She urged me to reconsider my relationship with wheat, as much of it is tainted with harmful pesticides. Her words resonated deeply, and I began to see the hidden dangers lurking in foods I had once considered safe.

As we delved into our discussions, she questioned my stance on Remicade, a medication often prescribed for my condition. I confessed my reservations, feeling that it was a suppressive measure rather than a genuine solution. Her response was a revelation: "I'm relieved you didn't choose Remicade. It doesn't heal; it merely suppresses. I'm disheartened by the rush to prescribe aggressive medications without giving our bodies a chance to heal naturally." We both nodded in agreement, acknowledging the limitations of conventional medicine.

We even shared a moment of humor, speculating that perhaps doctors had vested interests in companies like Johnson & Johnson, the manufacturer of Remicade. It was a lighthearted way of coping with the frustration we felt.

My journey led me to the concept of the elimination diet, a practice I was familiar with but had never truly embraced. It opened my eyes to the vast realm of nutritional knowledge hidden within the pages of history. Back in the 1940s through the 1980s, pioneers of natural and alternative medicine were uncovering the power of food in preventing and treating diseases.

I stumbled upon the work of Roger Williams, an American biochemist, whose book "Biochemical Individuality" emphasized the uniqueness of each person's metabolic makeup and micronutrient needs. It shattered the one-size-fits-all approach to nutrition, revealing that our bodies have distinct requirements.

For those intrigued by controversial figures, there was Dr. Sebi, a herbalist shunned by the Western medical community but who offered valuable insights. He resorted to researching the effects of nutrients from food. What he discovered was that nutrients from food had a remarkable ability to reduce inflammation, which, in turn, could influence gene expression and disease. Yet, much of this knowledge remains buried in research articles, overlooked in mainstream education.

The Elimination Diet

The elimination diet became my gateway to better health. It meant embracing a disciplined, nutritious diet while systematically reintroducing foods to identify adverse reactions and triggers for my condition. The process was meticulous but enlightening.

1. Proteins (Highly Encourage Whole Plant-Based Diet): I

learned to seek out lean, free-range, grass-fed, and organic sources like fish, poultry, and wild game while avoiding challenge foods like beef and processed meats. I also discovered the immense benefits of a whole plant-based diet, where foods like legumes, nuts, and seeds became my primary sources of protein during remission.

2. Legumes: I welcomed organic non-GMO legumes, especially after soaking them to remove indigestible sugars.

3. Nuts and Seeds: I embraced unsweetened, organic varieties, but took caution with some like peanuts, as they could be reintroduced later.

4. Oils and Fats: Cold-pressed, organic oils like olive oil and avocado oil became my allies, while I avoided inflammatory culprits like canola oil and margarine.

5. Dairy Alternatives: Organic and unsweetened options like almond and coconut milk took the place of conventional dairy.

6. Vegetables and Fruits: My plate was now filled with a colorful array of fresh vegetables and fruits, but I had to be mindful of the Dirty Dozen list, which highlighted pesticide-laden produce to buy organic.

7. Gluten-Free Grains: My grains of choice were amaranth, brown rice, and quinoa, while I waved goodbye to wheat, barley, and rye.

Starting the elimination diet was a journey in itself. Each food reintroduction was a careful experiment, and I had to note any adverse reactions over a two-day period. It was essential to stimulate my vagus nerve for better digestion and enjoy each bite, all while taking a deep breath to activate the parasympathetic nervous system. If a food provoked symptoms, it was eliminated, to be reintroduced at a later time.

The challenge foods like wheat, dairy, soy, and others were scrutinized for their effects on my body. I had the choice to avoid them indefinitely, knowing they had played a part in triggering inflammation.

But my journey didn't stop at elimination; it extended into the realm of anti-inflammatory foods. I discovered that fresh vegetables and fruits, particularly those rich in omega-3 fats, held the power to soothe inflammation. Extra virgin olive oil, and a diverse range of spices became staples in my diet. Dark leafy greens and colorful produce were my allies in the battle against inflammation.

In the end, my journey to health wasn't just about making great food choices; it was about uncovering the hidden potential within each meal and harnessing it to heal my body. It's a journey that continues, and I invite you to explore this path to wellness for yourself.

The Vital Role of a Whole Food Plant-Based Diet

One of the most transformative revelations during my journey was the realization of the importance of a whole food plant-based diet. This paradigm shift opened my eyes to the profound implications of our dietary choices.

I understood that meats, while traditionally consumed by many, could be acidic, placing stress on vital organs such as the adrenals, kidneys, and the lymphatic system. Moreover, they had the potential to contribute to mucus formation within the body. This profound insight encouraged me to explore plant-based alternatives that not only nourished the body but also harmonized with its natural processes.

The Journey Continues

My journey towards wellness wasn't a narrative of dietary shifts; it was an exploration of the healing power of food and the innate potential within our bodies to overcome adversity. This voyage persists, an ongoing quest to embrace the wisdom of alternative medicine, integrate whole food plant-based nutrition, and harmonize with the body's innate capacity to heal.

In this enduring journey, I extend an invitation to all those who seek wellness and vitality, a journey illuminated by the profound influence of dietary choices. It's an odyssey I encourage you to embark upon, for it leads to the transformative power of food and a path to a life of well-being and balance.

Chapter 17: Decoding Food Labels and Steering Clear of Additives

I n my nursing school days, we embarked on a mission to enhance senior citizens' health awareness. We visited senior centers, measuring vital signs and even joining seniors on their shopping trips, with the goal of promoting healthier eating habits. These elderly individuals often struggled to decipher food labels and grappled with pricing. Their gratitude and joy for our assistance were immeasurable.

It was during a project presentation for these seniors that I chose to demystify the art of reading labels. Many of the seniors, despite their wisdom, confessed that they'd lived for more than six decades on this planet without truly understanding what some of those cryptic food label terms meant. My presentation aimed to make it all simpler.

Unmasking the Deception: Front-of-Package Claims

Before we embark on the journey of deciphering nutrition information panel, there's one critical piece of advice: ignore the alluring claims on the front of the packaging. Those enticing labels often try to lure you into believing that the product is a healthy choice. But, the reality is, these claims are typically designed to mislead consumers and entice them into making a purchase.

These claims are nothing but clever marketing tactics aimed at convincing you that the product is a great choice for your health. Next time you encounter such marketing wizardry, know that you're onto their game. Remember, the first lesson in label reading is to disregard these front-of-package claims.

The Heart of Label Reading: Nutritional Facts and Ingredients

When it comes to deciphering food labels, the nutritional facts and ingredients list are your guiding stars. The nutritional facts provide valuable information about the nutrient content per serving, helping you make informed dietary choices. However, the real treasure lies in the ingredients list.

- Ingredients List Hierarchy: Ingredients are listed in order of quantity. The first ingredient is what manufacturers use most of, and as you move down the list, you encounter ingredients in descending order of proportion. Be keen to scrutinize this list because it reveals which components dominate the product.
- The Long Ingredient Lists Warning: Be skeptical when you spot a long list of ingredients. A plethora of additives, preservatives, and unpronounceable components often characterize these products. Such extensive lists should raise red flags and serve as an indicator to stay away.
- The Unknown Ingredients Trap: If you come across an ingredient you can't pronounce or have never heard of, it's probably a preservative or additive. These mysterious additives can be linked to inflammatory properties, making them a potential threat to your health.

Deciphering Serving Sizes: Beware the Illusion

One of the trickiest aspects of food labels is serving sizes. It's surprising to learn that many of these serving sizes are considerably smaller than what people consume in one sitting. This manipulation often leads to misleading interpretations of the food's nutritional content.

For instance, a chocolate bar might be labeled as having two servings. This forces consumers to double the calories and nutritional values in the nutritional facts for a more accurate representation of their consumption. Additionally, when a food item contains less than 0.5 grams of a particular nutrient, it can legally be reported as 0. This intriguing aspect results in deceptive labeling.

The Danger Zone: Additives and Preservatives

Navigating food labels also involves a cautious exploration of additives and preservatives. Many of these synthetic compounds are commonly used in processed foods, and they have garnered attention for their potential health risks. Some additives to be wary of include:

- Monosodium Glutamate (MSG): While MSG enhances the flavor of food, it can cause sensitivities in some individuals. Studies have shown that it is generally safe when used in moderation.
- Sodium Nitrite: This additive acts as a preservative, primarily used in meats to prevent bacterial growth and provide a reddish-pink color. The concern arises when sodium nitrate is heated at high temperatures, leading to the formation of nitrosamines, which are carcinogenic.
- Artificial Food Coloring: These colorful additives are used

to brighten foods, but their safety has been debated for decades. Some animal studies have linked high doses of food dyes to organ damage, cancer, and birth defects. Behavioral issues in children have also been associated with food dyes.

- Guar Gum: Derived from guar beans, this polysaccharide has thickening and stabilizing properties. While it has benefits, excessive consumption can lead to intestinal blockage.
- High-Fructose Corn Syrup: Used as a sweetener in foods and beverages, excessive intake of high-fructose corn syrup has been linked to various health problems, including obesity and insulin resistance.
- Carrageenan: Derived from red seaweed, it acts as a thickener and preservative in foods. Some studies suggest that carrageenan may contribute to high blood sugar and intestinal ulcers. More research is needed to confirm these findings.
- Artificial Sweeteners: The five artificial sweeteners approved by the FDA are sucralose, saccharin, acesulfame, aspartame, and neotame. These intensely sweet compounds can influence the way the human body responds to sweetness, potentially affecting food preferences.
- Sodium Benzoate: As a preservative, sodium benzoate, when combined with vitamin C, can form benzene, a compound with potential carcinogenic properties.
- Trans Fats: These unsaturated fats, created through hydrogenation, are found in products like margarine and microwave popcorn. Trans fats have been linked to health issues, including inflammation and heart disease.

In conclusion, it's crucial to limit or eliminate these additives and preservatives from your diet. These recommendations are based on cautious vigilance rather than concrete scientific certainty. Our bodies remain complex, and there's much we're yet to fully comprehend. However, eliminating these potentially harmful substances has profoundly impacted my health, restoring a life free from the debilitating symptoms that once plagued me. Remember, life is a precious gift, and our health is the most valuable treasure we possess. Health truly is wealth, far more precious than silver and gold. It's a gift to cherish, nurture, and protect for ourselves and the generations that follow.

Chapter 18: Embracing a Lifestyle, Not Just a Diet: The Mediterranean Way

The term "diet" has become laden with negative connotations. It often conjures images of restriction, temporary fixes, and, more often than not, leads to frustration and ultimate failure. The time has come to liberate ourselves from the unending cycle of dieting and instead embark on a journey of a lifelong lifestyle change. This change focuses on nourishing the body from within, with a foundation built upon whole plant-based foods, offering a healthier alternative to meat, such as fish.

The Mediterranean diet, often hailed as a blueprint for healthy living, encapsulates the essence of this lifestyle. At its core, it revolves around the consumption of foods like fruits, vegetables, nuts, and whole grains. Additionally, it encourages the inclusion of whole plant-based options such as legumes and tofu. Fish, a staple of this diet, is considered a fantastic source of lean protein and is abundant in essential omega-3 fatty acids.

To make this dietary shift, consider integrating fish into your meals once a week, especially those varieties rich in omega-3 fatty acids. Salmon, mackerel, herring, and sardines are among the top choices due to their high content of these essential fats. While other types of fish can also be included, prioritize wild-caught options for their superior nutritional value. If you opt for farmed fish, be discerning in your choice and select fish from countries with stringent regulations, such as the USA, Norway, and Australia.

Fish is not merely a source of lean protein; it is also a treasure trove of vital nutrients, including vitamin D. Its light and easily digestible nature make it an excellent dietary choice, and it offers a myriad of health benefits. However, this journey isn't solely about fish; it encompasses a broader spectrum of foods.

One particular category of fruits that we should explore in our pursuit of wellness is the group of astringent fruits. These fruits include grapes, oranges, apples, mangoes, pineapples, and limes. With their high water content and the ability to cleanse and soothe our digestive systems, pulling mucus out of the body, they are crucial in our journey toward health.

As we delve deeper into this lifestyle, it's vital to acknowledge the immense contributions of antioxidants present in these fruits. These compounds are our allies, safeguarding our cells against oxidative stress, thus reducing inflammation and diminishing the risk of chronic diseases. They serve as a refreshing and essential component on our path to robust health.

The time has come to liberate ourselves from the constraints of conventional diets. It's time to embrace a way of eating that not only nourishes but also heals. This is more than just a diet; it's a lifelong commitment to your well-being. The Mediterranean diet, enriched by the inclusion of phytonutrient-rich fruits like melons and cucumbers, acts as your guiding star on this profound journey. Say goodbye to the limitations of dieting and welcome a life filled with robust health and unwavering vitality.

Let me emphasize how transformative dietary practices can be for one's health. My experience is a testament to the significant improvement that can result from a well-thought-out diet. My journey, marked by positive changes evident in subsequent medical assessments like colonoscopies, showcases the power of adopting a mindful and health-focused approach to eating.

Chapter 19: Unearthing Allergies

Off I went to see the allergist, with high hopes of uncovering potential food intolerances. To my surprise, the allergist clarified that her expertise lay in allergic reactions rather than food intolerances. Nonetheless, my allergies, which included seasonal allergies and shellfish seafood-induced lip swelling and rashes, did capture her interest. We even delved into my previous reaction to Penicillin, which, surprisingly, had not repeated when I was administered Rocephin in the hospital.

In an effort to gain further insight into these allergies, I steeled myself for the experience of enduring 47 needle shots in my back, along with a histamine control. The verdict was in: I was indeed allergic to trees, grass, and weeds, in addition to cats and Penicillin. However, the intriguing part was that my body seemed to harbor no grudge against seafood. This revelation was later solidified through blood tests. While these allergies tests were informative, they did not provide insight as to whether or not I had ulcerative colitis.

Chapter 20: A Glimmer of Hope

M onths of steadfast lifestyle changes culminated in a pivotal moment: my scheduled endoscopy and colonoscopy. The daunting prep with Miralax and Dulcolax was a thunderous prologue. I enlisted my dad as my chauffeur and, in the parking lot, we enjoyed some quality bonding time, his wisdom always a source of inspiration.

At the hospital, I went through the customary check-in and an engaging conversation with a nurse who was impressed by my prominent veins. The IV setup was swift, and I found myself in the procedure room.

Under sedation, my memory turned hazy. However, the outcomes were far from vague. Remarkably, inflammation had dwindled, leaving only mild traces in my sigmoid colon – a dormant state of my ulcerative colitis. The word "remission" danced in the air, and I was jubilant. My endoscopy hinted at mild gastritis, a bump in the road that lifestyle changes would eventually smooth out.

As my doctor approved the reduction in my Colazal dosage, I eagerly anticipated the days ahead. After the EGD (Esophagog astroduodenoscopy) and colonoscopy, I have been diagnosed with ulcerative pancolitis without complication, a form of ulcerative colitis that affects the entire large intestine, I've diligently followed my current regimen. My GI doctor strongly recommended it due to its apparent success.

Chapter 21: A Day in the Life of Resilience

Each day dawns with a ritual that symbolizes the embodiment of a holistic and resilient lifestyle. My mornings begin with an obligatory visit to the porcelain throne, a humbling reminder of the body's natural processes. Following this routine, I ingest a tablespoon of extra virgin olive oil on an empty stomach, igniting a sequence of choices and practices that are the cornerstones of my well-being.

The first challenge of the day is breakfast. It's not merely a meal but an opportunity to nourish both myself and my children with a purposeful and health-driven selection of dishes. My commitment extends to a regimented intake of essential supplements, ensuring that our bodies receive the nutrients necessary for optimal functioning.

The heart of my daily life revolves around a rigorous strength training regimen that touches every major muscle group. This commitment to exercise includes dedicated sessions for the chest, back, legs, triceps, biceps, and shoulders, each meticulously planned to achieve a sense of balance. To complement the strength training, a sprinkle of cardio and yoga sessions rounds out the exercise routine, addressing not only physical strength but also mental and emotional equilibrium.

Post-workout, the body requires replenishment, and I answer this need with a combination of collagen peptides and organic aloe vera juice. These choices represent my conscious effort to provide the body with the tools to recover and thrive. Following this post-workout phase, the focus shifts to spending precious quality time with my son. It's a vital connection that strengthens both our emotional bonds and our resilience.

My commitment to a healthy lifestyle extends to meal preparation. The process is meticulous, involving careful planning, vacuum-sealing, and freezing. These efforts are underpinned by a conscious choice to favor the stove or toaster oven over the microwave, eliminating potential health risks and retaining the nutritional value of our meals.

The shared family lunches are not just meals; they are moments of togetherness that I cherish. They serve as a reminder of the fleeting nature of time and the importance of nurturing relationships that form the foundation of our lives.

As the day unfolds, I engage in deep breathing techniques that help center my body and mind. These practices are designed to alleviate stress, instill focus, and reinforce my resolve. A series of introspective questions follows, aimed at identifying and conquering self-defeating thoughts and barriers that may threaten my emotional well-being.

Reflecting on Self-Talk:

- What thoughts dominate my mind when facing challenges?
- Are these thoughts empowering or self-defeating?
- How can I reframe negative thoughts into positive affirmations?

Analyzing Emotional Triggers:

- What situations or interactions trigger stress or negative emotions?
- How can I respond differently to these triggers in a more positive way?
- Are there patterns in my emotional responses that I can address?

Examining Limiting Beliefs:

- What beliefs about myself might be holding me back?
- Are these beliefs based on reality or unfounded assumptions?
- How can I challenge and change limiting beliefs that hinder my well-being?

Goal Setting and Progress:

- What are my short-term and long-term goals for emotional well-being?
- What steps can I take today to move closer to these goals?
- How can I celebrate and acknowledge my progress, no matter how small?

Practicing Gratitude:

- What aspects of my life am I grateful for right now?
- How can I incorporate gratitude into my daily routine?
- How does focusing on gratitude shift my perspective and mindset?

Cultivating Self-Compassion:

- How do I talk to myself when I make mistakes or face challenges?
- Can I offer myself the same kindness and understanding I would give to a friend?
- What self-compassionate affirmations can I use to counteract self-criticism?

Remember, these questions are tools for self-reflection and personal growth. The goal is to foster a deeper understanding of oneself and to develop strategies for maintaining emotional well-being in the face of life's challenges.

The evening is a realm of cherished moments with my two boys. It is a space where we bond, learn, and grow together. These precious moments culminate in their bedtime routine, where stories, laughter, and love are abundant.

The final act of the day is dedicated to personal relaxation and indulgence in mindless activities. It's a vital part of unwinding and maintaining balance. As the day comes to a close, I conclude with the nightly intake of probiotics, a soothing warm shower, and well-deserved rest. These practices form the foundation of a restorative night, ensuring I wake up ready to face the challenges and opportunities of a new day.

This daily ritual is a testament to my unwavering commitment to a healthy life. It is a path I've chosen to tread, one that leads me through adversity and towards the resilience needed to embrace each day with hope and purpose.

Chapter 22: The Hematologist's Verdict

It all began on the day etched in my memory when I noticed the alarming changes in my right leg, the source of my distress. This unusual warmth and persistent redness in my leg sent shockwaves of concern through my being. The urgency of the situation led me to seek medical attention. I scheduled a visit with my primary physician, who recognized the gravity of the situation and acted promptly.

The primary physician initiated this journey of medical exploration and answers. A critical step in this quest for clarity was a thorough evaluation of my leg. The initial examinations and discussions culminated in a pivotal moment – the second ultrasound that would unveil the underlying issue. Their results were as undeniable as they were concerning – a blood clot was discovered in my right leg.

With this diagnosis came the prescription for Xarelto, a blood thinner. It was a significant intervention meant to address this emergent medical issue, and it initiated a 90-day treatment regimen. It was a path riddled with uncertainty, the weight of which I bore during those days of treatment. Every dosage of Xarelto, an assurance of my commitment to my own well-being, came with the hope that it would bring me closer to a life free from the shackles of this condition.

With each passing day, the completion of the 90-day course drew nearer. It was a period marked by hope and concern, a period in which I had to grapple with the complex interplay between medication and recovery. My anxieties were quelled by a crucial examination – the d-dimer test. This was a vital measurement, a tool that medical professionals used to rule out harmful blood clots and gauge the effectiveness of the treatment.

The moment of truth arrived as the hematologist reviewed my case. This medical expert, with profound knowledge of blood disorders, would hold the key to my path forward. As my history and test results were laid bare, a unanimous decision began to crystallize.

The consensus was clear – there was no need for me to continue the anticoagulation therapy. I did not exhibit the presence of other triggers for blood clots, and this was, in fact, my first episode. The timing of the blood clot's emergence, one week after my hospital discharge, hinted at the possibility that severe dehydration had rendered me more susceptible to this condition. This conclusion was a silver lining that I had yearned for. It was an assurance that my perseverance was leading me down the right path.

With the hematologist's verdict echoing in my ears, the decision was made. No further blood work or treatment adjustments were required. The parting words of my encounter with this specialist carry an unforgettable charm. I turned to him, my relief evident in my eyes, and said, "You seem like a cool guy, but I hope I'll never see you again. Are you okay with that?" A hearty laugh and an approving nod were his response, and we parted ways.

For me, this was a pivotal moment. It was the assurance I needed to step forward with renewed determination in my pursuit of health. As I bid farewell to the hematologist, the weight of one less medication on my daily roster was palpable. It was an opportunity to reset, recommit, and continue the journey with newfound hope and vigor.

Chapter 23: Recipes and Regimen – The Holistic Harmony

In the preceding chapters, we've embarked on a journey of self-discovery and health transformation. We've explored the intricacies of the human body, unraveling the complexities of medical conditions, and navigating the labyrinth of dietary choices. It's been a quest for truth, a search for well-being, and a commitment to holistic health.

Now, it's time to weave all this knowledge into a holistic tapestry of well-being. This chapter unveils a simple yet flexible plan, a practical blueprint for readers, to help you achieve vibrant health and allow room for personal adjustments. I'll emphasize the pivotal role of meal preparation as the linchpin of success and provide you with a strategy to keep you on track, staving off those times when hunger strikes and the fridge remains disappointingly bare. The secret? Embrace the vacuum sealer and a well-stocked freezer, and we'll show you how.

In this holistic regimen, calorie restriction takes a backseat, for the true aim is to recalibrate the body's balance. I'll introduce a visual cue that will guide your plate assembly – envision a rainbow. As you prepare your meals, ensure a palette of colors that mirrors nature's bounty. This isn't just about aesthetics; it's about providing your body with a diverse array of nutrients.

To bring balance to your microbiome, you'll make friends with fermented foods. The western diet, often dominated by processed fare, starves our good gut bacteria. Fermented foods, from beans to kimchi, stand as nature's replenishing agents for a diverse microbiome. We'll explore the world of fermentation and show you how to incorporate these gut-friendly foods into your daily life.

But there's more to holistic well-being than just gut health. We'll delve into the profound impact of diet on mucus in the human body. By consuming foods that are inherently designed for the human vessel, we can mitigate mucus production. You'll discover how mucus acts as the body's safeguard against the corrosive influence of foreign substances, including acid-forming foods. It often harbors toxins, locks in metals and chemicals, and provides a fertile breeding ground for yeast, fungi, and parasites.

We'll reveal the fruits that lead the charge in eradicating mucus. Foods like citrus, grapes, apples, grapefruit and mangoes play a crucial role in facilitating mucus expulsion. You'll learn how to incorporate these mucus-busting foods into your diet, harnessing their cleansing power for improved well-being.

Vegetable matter, particularly chlorophyll-rich green drinks, serves a different but equally vital role. These green beverages act as brooms, sweeping away mucus and biofilm from the colon's outer layer. We'll show you how to include these detoxifying green drinks in your daily routine.

In your holistic health journey, you'll also explore the world of an all-fruit diet as a potent detoxifying agent. This diet drains the body of debris and metabolic waste, helping you rebuild after the damaging effects of acidic foods. Fruits emerge as the body's trusted cleaners, assisting you in expelling mucus and toxins.

As the chapter unfolds, readers are encouraged to harness the inherent vitality of fruits, exploring the magical world of detoxification and discovering how they can rebuild the body. You'll learn the hidden secrets of an all-fruit diet, guiding you toward cleansing, rebuilding, and unlocking your body's incredible potential.

Mucus's days are numbered in the presence of high-energy, astringent foods. Fruits will emerge as the key to your holistic health journey, guiding you toward renewed well-being and vitality. It's time to set yourself free from the shackles of mucus and acid-forming foods, charting a path to lasting health.

Chapter 24: The Unveiling Power of Functional Medicine

A s my health journey continued to unfold, it led me to an enlightening realm: Functional Medicine. I did see a Functional Medicine Specialist and this transformative approach marked a significant turning point in my quest to regain my well-being and become the healthiest version of myself. In this chapter, I'll take you on a guided tour of what functional medicine is, how it played a pivotal role in my story, and why you should consider it too.

The Discovery of Functional Medicine

Functional Medicine is a patient-centered approach to healthcare that transcends the boundaries of mere symptom management. It seeks to address the underlying causes of illness, offering a comprehensive, personalized approach tailored to each patient's unique health concerns. It combines the best aspects of conventional medicine with a holistic, integrative perspective that takes into account the individual's lifestyle, genetics, and environment.

Unmasking the Mold Mystery

For me, the journey into Functional Medicine began when

a comprehensive stool study taken when I visited Functional Medicine Specialist uncovered a startling revelation: my body was playing host to an abnormally high amount of mold. Dysbiosis, a gut condition marked by an imbalance of good and bad bacteria, had taken root in my system, causing a myriad of health issues. While this discovery was undoubtedly disconcerting, it didn't fully explain how I'd become a host to these unwelcome microbes.

The real eureka moment came when I traced my exposure back to my workplace. It turned out that my previous job had unknowingly been a hub for mold infestation. This knowledge dawned upon me before I even began my new role in a different location. It was a startling revelation that linked my health struggles to environmental factors.

The Clue: Petri Dish Test

To give credence to my suspicions, I embarked on a simple yet revealing experiment. I conducted a Petri dish test at the workplace, leaving the dish exposed in the suspected contaminated area for just one hour. What it revealed was nothing short of shocking – over 17 dangerous mold colonies had rapidly established themselves. This was the missing puzzle piece, the cause of my persistent health problems and the key to understanding my struggles.

A total of 10 employees confirmed the findings of mold at the workplace. Only one colleague and I underwent testing; he was dealing with his health issues and tested positive for high amounts of mold.

The Genetic Key: HLA-DR/DQ Testing

An integral component of my Functional Medicine journey

was the HLA-DR/DQ genetic test. This test uncovered a fundamental aspect of my health struggle: my body's inability to effectively rid itself of mold toxins. The test showed that I carried genetic markers associated with reduced mold detoxification capabilities. This genetic predisposition had paved the way for high levels of inflammation, my immune system attacking my own body, and an excess of troublesome mucus.

The Promise of Functional Medicine

Functional Medicine, with its focus on personalized, root-cause treatment, offered a glimmer of hope on the horizon. Instead of suppressing symptoms, it aimed to treat the core issues that had been plaguing my health. It meant addressing my mold exposure and finding effective ways to detoxify my system. I embarked on a transformative journey of lifestyle adjustments, dietary modifications, targeted supplements, and detox protocols.

The path ahead was not without its challenges, but with Functional Medicine guiding the way, I finally began to see the light at the end of the tunnel. Gradually, I regained my health, managed my inflammation, and witnessed my body recover from its self-attacking tendencies. The excessive mucus production that had plagued me for so long began to subside.

Why Functional Medicine?

Functional Medicine is not just my story; it's an approach that holds immense promise for anyone grappling with chronic health issues. It provides a holistic framework, addressing your body as a complex, interconnected system. It doesn't merely treat your symptoms; it investigates their origins. By focusing on your unique genetic makeup, lifestyle, and environmental factors, Functional Medicine offers a tailored, comprehensive solution.

In the following chapters, I'll delve into the specific details of my Functional Medicine journey, sharing the practical steps I took and the positive changes I experienced. The story of my health transformation through this approach serves as a testament to the potential it holds for anyone ready to take the reins of their well-being. Together, we'll explore how Functional Medicine can become your partner on the path to optimal health and vitality.

Chapter 25: The Hero's Odyssey to Detoxification

I n the grand tapestry of my health journey, this chapter shines as a testament to the indomitable spirit of the human body, the power of determination, and the wisdom of Functional Medicine. This stage of my quest was characterized by battles fought not with swords, but with knowledge and persistence. Let me take you on a journey through the labyrinth of detoxification, revealing the transformational role of charcoal, Bentonite clay, and N-acetylcysteine (NAC) in purging the lurking demons within.

The Mold Menace

Mold – a seemingly innocuous, ever-present entity that, in my case, morphed into a relentless adversary. My health had been held hostage by molds that had covertly invaded my system. These weren't the commonplace molds that often appear on a forgotten loaf of bread or the shower curtain; they were the high-contrast, dangerous molds capable of causing immense harm to the human body.

Dangers Lurking in the Shadows

Mold, when left unchecked, can unleash an array of health

horrors. It's not just a matter of the unpleasant smell or the unsightly patches that sometimes adorn our living spaces. Dangerous molds, like the notorious Stachybotrys, Aspergillus, or Penicillium, produce mycotoxins – chemical byproducts that can wreak havoc on our health. Exposure to these toxins can lead to a myriad of health problems, including respiratory issues, fatigue, chronic sinusitis, brain fog, and even more severe conditions.

In my case, mold had infiltrated my body and induced a prolonged battle with inflammation, immune system dysregulation, and an unrelenting production of mucous. My health had been besieged, and it was time to mount a defense.

The Detox Arsenal

Armed with the knowledge of Functional Medicine and guided by a skilled practitioner, I embarked on a challenging journey of detoxification. My quest involved a multifaceted approach to purging my system of these unwelcome intruders, where charcoal, Bentonite clay, and NAC became my allies.

Charcoal: The Black Elixir

Activated charcoal, a dark and enigmatic substance, is a potent detoxification tool. Its porous structure is adept at absorbing a variety of impurities, including mycotoxins. This "black elixir" became a crucial part of my daily regimen.

By introducing activated charcoal into my detox routine, I effectively initiated a process known as adsorption (not to be confused with absorption). It acted like a magnet, binding mycotoxins and other harmful substances to its surface. My body could then safely eliminate these captives through the usual routes, such as urine and feces.

Bentonite Clay: Nature's Cleansing Agent

Bentonite clay, known as "healing clay," proved to be another formidable detoxification agent. This natural substance, formed from volcanic ash, contains powerful negatively charged ions. When consumed, it attracts and binds to positively charged toxins, drawing them out of the body.

Through regular use of Bentonite clay, I was able to systematically free my system from the grasp of mycotoxins. Its gentle but effective cleansing properties made it an invaluable addition to my detox regimen.

NAC: The Glutathione Booster

N-acetyl cysteine (NAC), a lesser-known hero in the detoxification journey, plays a critical role in supporting the body's master antioxidant, glutathione. Glutathione is the body's primary defense mechanism against mycotoxins and other toxins. However, my battle-weary body had a deficiency in this vital antioxidant.

By incorporating NAC into my routine, I was effectively boosting my glutathione levels. This allowed my body to more efficiently neutralize and eliminate the lingering mycotoxins. NAC proved to be a potent ally in my quest for detoxification and recovery.

The Culmination of Years

This process of detoxification was no quick fix. It was a patient, relentless pursuit that spanned years. The impact of detoxification doesn't manifest overnight. It's a gradual unfolding of better health, driven by consistent and mindful practices.

A Comprehensive Approach to Mold

But it wasn't only the internal detoxification that played a role. Another pivotal move was addressing the source of my mold exposure. I took proactive steps to reach out to my workplace, urging them to address the mold infestation that had cast a shadow over my health.

Their immediate response in cleaning up the mold was a beacon of hope. It underscored the importance of advocating for one's health and safety. Understanding the dangers of mold and actively working to eliminate its presence is a crucial aspect of any detoxification journey.

A Never-Ending Vigilance

The battle against mold isn't one that can ever truly be declared victorious. Mold is an ever-present entity in our environment. It's a reminder that we must remain vigilant in safeguarding our health.

But my journey illuminated the path towards a healthier, mold-resilient life. It also underscored the invaluable role of functional medicine, where individualized approaches to health can lead to remarkable transformations.

Chapter 26: Diving into Detoxification

In the course of our journey, we've delved into the depths of Functional Medicine, braving treacherous terrain, vanquishing health adversaries, and unlocking the secrets of holistic healing. With the foundations firmly laid, it's time to equip you with the practical tools for detoxification. This chapter serves as the treasure trove of protocols and strategies that I personally followed on my quest to optimal health.

Fasting

Fasting, particularly a 24-hour dry fast or a 3-4 day water fast with the addition of Celtic salt, sea salt, or Himalayan salt (as opposed to table salt), has pique my interest because of its potential effects on my health, particularly in promoting autophagy, stem cell production, human growth hormone (HGH) release,cellular repair, mold and parasite removal detoxification and digestive rest. Let me elaborate on these aspects:

1. Autophagy: I've learned that autophagy is a fascinating process where my body removes damaged or dysfunctional cellular components to enhance overall cellular health. The idea that fasting can trigger autophagy intrigues me. It's like my body starts spring cleaning when

I deprive it of nutrients for a while, breaking down and recycling old or damaged cellular parts.

2. Stem Cell Production: The concept that fasting can boost the production of stem cells is intriguing. Stem cells have the potential to regenerate different types of cells in my body, potentially contributing to tissue repair and regeneration. This has implications for my overall health and well-being.

3. HGH Release: I've learned that fasting, especially during extended periods, can stimulate the release of human growth hormone (HGH). HGH plays a crucial role in growth, metabolism, and overall health. The thought that fasting can lead to increased HGH levels is appealing because it could potentially help with fat loss, muscle preservation, and more.

4. Cellular Repair: I find it fascinating that fasting can promote cellular repair processes. When I'm fasting, my body shifts its focus from digestion to repair and maintenance. This includes repairing DNA, synthesizing proteins, and eliminating damaged cellular components through autophagy.

5. Mold and Parasite Removal: I've learned that fasting can create an environment in the body that is less conducive to the survival of mold and parasites. These microorganisms thrive in the presence of food, and fasting deprives them of their primary source of sustenance. As a result, fasting may help in reducing the population of mold and parasites in my body, potentially leading to improved gut health and overall well-being.

6. Detoxification: Fasting is often associated with detoxification processes in the body. The increased metabolic

activity during fasting, combined with the removal of toxins through various pathways, can assist in cleansing the body. This can lead to a feeling of increased vitality and overall health.

7. Digestive Rest: Fasting also provides a break for the digestive system. This period of rest allows the digestive organs to recuperate and can contribute to the expulsion of waste and toxins, which may include parasites and mold that have accumulated in the digestive tract.

As for the choice of salt during fasting, I've come to understand that Celtic salt, sea salt, and Himalayan salt are often preferred over table salt due to their natural and less processed nature. These salts contain essential minerals that can help maintain electrolyte balance during a fast, reducing the risk of dehydration and other potential side effects.

However, it's essential to remember that fasting is a highly individualized experience, and the effects can vary from person to person based on factors like age, overall health, and diet. Fasting is not a one-size-fits-all approach.

In my journey, I'm aware of the risks associated with fasting, especially during extended periods, and I'm committed to approaching it with caution. I understand the importance of consulting with a healthcare professional before embarking on any fasting regimen, especially considering my unique circumstances and health status.

Ultimately, while fasting presents intriguing potential health benefits, it's crucial for me to approach it mindfully and make well-informed decisions based on my individual goals and circumstances.

Understanding Parasites

Parasites are organisms that live in or on another organism (the host) and benefit at the host's expense. In the context of human health, parasites can take many forms, including protozoa, helminths (worms), and ectoparasites like ticks and mites. Contrary to popular belief, parasites are not limited to tropical or underdeveloped regions; they can affect people worldwide. Parasites, the often overlooked inhabitants of our bodies, can cause a range of health issues that might surprise many. They can create backups in our lymphatic system, starve us of essential minerals, and even lead to constipation.

Effects of Parasites on the Body

Parasites can wreak havoc on the human body, causing a range of detrimental effects. They can disrupt the digestive system, leading to symptoms such as diarrhea, nausea, and abdominal pain. Some parasites migrate to other organs, causing inflammation and damage. In severe cases, parasites can lead to malnutrition, anemia, and weakened immunity, leaving individuals vulnerable to secondary infections. Certain parasites can even affect the nervous system, causing neurological symptoms. Overall, the presence of parasites can significantly impair physical health and overall well-being, highlighting the importance of prevention and treatment measures.

Lymphatic System Backup

Parasites can impede the proper functioning of our lymphatic system, a crucial part of our immune and circulatory systems. The lymphatic system is responsible for carrying white blood cells, removing waste and toxins, and maintaining fluid balance in the body. When parasites infect this system, they can disrupt these functions, leading to issues like swelling and fluid retention.

Mineral Depletion

Parasites can also be "mineral thieves." They consume essential minerals in the body, such as iron, magnesium, and calcium, leaving the host deficient. Mineral deficiencies can result in a range of symptoms, from fatigue and muscle weakness to problems with bone health.

Digestive Problems

Many people suffering from parasitic infections report digestive problems, including constipation, diarrhea, and abdominal pain. These issues often arise due to the parasites' interference with the gastrointestinal tract.

Functional Medicine and Parasite Removal

Functional medicine is an approach to healthcare that seeks to identify and address the root causes of illness. When it comes to parasites, functional medicine recognizes the importance of parasite cleansing to restore and maintain overall health.

Common Parasite Cleansing Methods
Black Walnut

Black walnut is a popular herbal remedy known for its anti-parasitic properties. It contains compounds like juglone, which can help eliminate parasites from the body.

Wormwood Herb

Wormwood is another potent herb often used in parasite cleansing. It contains compounds like artemisinin, which have been shown to be effective against various parasites.

Cat's Claw Bark

Cat's claw, a traditional herbal remedy, is known for its immune-boosting properties and may help combat parasites.

Wormseed Herb

Wormseed, as the name suggests, is used to eliminate worms and parasites in traditional medicine.

Cascara Sagrada Bark

Cascara sagrada is a natural laxative that can aid in eliminating parasites and promoting regular bowel movements.

Biocidin

Biocidin is a herbal complex containing various botanical ingredients with antimicrobial properties. It may support parasite cleansing

Pau d'Arco Bark

Pau d'Arco is an herbal remedy that may have anti-parasitic properties, particularly against fungi and yeast overgrowth.

Dietary Components

Certain foods like garlic, pumpkin seeds, and papaya seeds have been used traditionally to cleanse the body of parasites. These foods contain natural compounds that can help expel or kill parasites.

Additional Remedies

Other herbal remedies like barberry root, clove bud, tansy herb, and fennel seed are also used to target parasites and support digestive health.

Supporting Detoxification

While the above remedies can help eliminate parasites, it's crucial to support the detoxification process. Taking a binder, such as activated charcoal, pectin, silica, or zeolite, can be beneficial. These binders can help capture and remove toxins and waste products released by parasites during their elimination.

Common Symptoms During Parasite Cleansing

Parasite cleansing can sometimes lead to uncomfortable symptoms. Herxheimer reactions, also known as "die-off" reactions, can occur when the body eliminates a significant number of parasites. Symptoms can include headaches, fatigue, and gastrointestinal discomfort. These reactions are generally temporary and a sign that the body is ridding itself of parasites.

The Importance of Holistic Health

Parasite cleansing is just one part of maintaining holistic health. It's essential to adopt a balanced lifestyle that includes a nutritious diet, regular exercise, stress management, and good hygiene practices. Regular health check-ups can help identify and address potential health issues, including parasitic infections.

Parasites are a prevalent but often underestimated health concern that can lead to a range of issues, from lymphatic system disruptions to mineral deficiencies and digestive problems. Recognizing the importance of cleansing and adopting a functional medicine approach can help individuals regain their health and well-being. With a variety of herbal remedies and detoxification methods available, addressing parasites can be a significant step towards a healthier life. However, it's important to consult with healthcare professionals and take a holistic approach to health and wellness

The Power of Personalized Protocols

In the realm of Functional Medicine, the one-size-fits-all

approach is a relic of the past. The hallmark of this methodology is personalized care. By understanding that each individual is unique, we can tailor detoxification protocols to suit specific needs.

As a prologue to this practical journey, it's crucial to underscore the significance of working with a qualified Functional Medicine practitioner. Their expertise will help you navigate the complexities of detoxification, ensuring that your journey is safe, effective, and attuned to your body's needs.

The Detoxification Arsenal

1. Mycotoxin Binders: These compounds, including activated charcoal and Bentonite clay, have already been introduced in our previous chapter. They play a pivotal role in binding mycotoxins, rendering them harmless and facilitating their elimination from the body.

2. NAC and Glutathione: As allies in detoxification, N-acetyl cysteine (NAC) and glutathione deserve special mention. NAC supports the production of glutathione, our body's primary antioxidant, strengthening its ability to neutralize and eliminate toxins.

3. IV Therapy: Intravenous therapy, administered by a qualified healthcare professional, offers a rapid and efficient way to deliver detoxifying agents directly into the bloodstream. It's a powerful tool in cases where immediate intervention is required.

4. Detox Diets: Various detox diets, such as the ketogenic

diet and elimination diets, can be beneficial. They aim to reduce inflammation, eliminate triggers, and optimize the body's natural detox processes.

5. Nutrient Supplements: Specific nutrients, including vitamins, minerals, and antioxidants, can support the body's detox pathways. Vitamin C, glutathione, zinc, and magnesium are some examples.

6. Sauna Therapy: Sweating is a natural means of detoxification. Sauna therapy can accelerate this process by promoting the release of toxins through perspiration.

7. Exercise: Regular physical activity not only improves circulation but also supports the lymphatic system in flushing out waste and toxins. Choose a form of exercise that you enjoy, ensuring consistency.

8. Mindfulness and Stress Reduction: Emotional and psychological toxins can be equally detrimental. Mindfulness practices, meditation, and stress reduction techniques can help you declutter your mental landscape.

9. Hydration: Adequate hydration is essential for all detoxification pathways. It supports kidney and liver function, assisting in the removal of waste products.

10. Sleep: The body undergoes significant detoxification processes during deep sleep. Prioritize a good night's rest to support these vital functions.

Monitoring Progress

As you embark on your detoxification journey, it's essential to have measurable metrics to assess your progress. Functional Medicine practitioners may utilize various tests to evaluate the efficiency of detoxification processes. These tests include:

1. Mycotoxin Testing: Analyzing urine or blood samples can reveal the presence of mycotoxins, providing insight into your mold exposure.

2. Comprehensive Metabolic Panel: A blood test can assess your liver and kidney function, key players in detoxification.

3. Liver Detoxification Profile: By evaluating the function of specific liver enzymes, you can gain insights into the efficiency of your liver's detox pathways.

4. Genetic Testing: As seen in my case, genetic tests, such as HLA-DR/DQ, can provide valuable information about your body's predisposition to detoxify efficiently.

5. Gut Health Assessment: Your gastrointestinal health directly influences detoxification. Stool tests and gut function assessments can be revealing.

6. Inflammatory Markers: Evaluating inflammatory markers in the blood can indicate the effectiveness of your detox protocols.

7. Kidney Function Tests: Kidneys play a critical role in waste elimination. Monitoring kidney function is a vital part of tracking detox progress.

Conclusion:

The Continuation of the Journey: I am currently off all prescribed medications and have embraced a regimen of holistic supplements. I incorporate alkaline teas, Irish sea moss, ormus, and black seed oil into my routine. Moreover, excessive supplementation can disrupt the body's natural balance. For instance, taking high doses of one nutrient may interfere with the absorption or utilization of others, leading to nutritional imbalances. While I remain on the detox journey, I maintain a healthy diet and limit my supplementation. Occasionally, I take magnesium glycinate, vitamin D, and fish oil base of lab work. I eat mostly whole plant base. In the rare event of a potential flare-up, I immediately turn to Slippery Elm and Marshmallow Root on an empty stomach, without any other supplements or food.

In my battle with ulcerative colitis, setbacks were inevitable, but my misplaced confidence proved to be the greatest challenge. After experiencing periods of relative wellness, I allowed myself to believe I could return to the familiar comforts of my old habits. The illusion of invincibility led me down a treacherous path.

Nights spent indulging in alcohol and fast food seemed harmless at first, but the consequences were swift and severe. The temporary pleasure was swiftly overshadowed by the agonizing return of flares. It wasn't an immediate crash but a slow, insidious unraveling of my progress.

The heavy consumption of processed foods, once again, became my undoing. Each bite seemed innocent enough, but collectively they fueled the resurgence of debilitating symptoms. It was a harsh reminder that my body demanded more than mere convenience; it required nourishment and care.

Ulcerative colitis taught me the unforgiving truth: there are no shortcuts on the path to recovery. Every setback served as a stark reminder of the delicate balance between health and indulgence. But amidst the challenges, I found resilience. Each setback became a lesson, guiding me towards a newfound understanding of self-care and perseverance in the face of adversity.

As we conclude our exploration of Functional Medicine and detoxification, let this chapter be your compass and toolkit. Your path toward optimal health is a lifelong voyage guided by knowledge, personalization, and resilience.

Throughout the preceding chapters, I've shared my narrative and insights, hoping you find inspiration and practical guidance. The journey to health is seldom linear, but it is always worth the pursuit. Detoxification, as part of the Functional Medicine approach, represents a formidable weapon in your arsenal.

Chapter 27: Revitalize Your Health: The Vegan Lifestyle Unveiled

A s we conclude this transformative journey, let's delve even deeper into the profound realm of veganism as the ultimate detoxification for the human body. In the following extensive exploration, we'll scrutinize how adopting a vegan lifestyle, with a robust emphasis on fruits, becomes the key to unlocking your body's innate detoxification potential.

A Paradigm Shift: The Detoxifying Power of Veganism

The journey towards optimal health demands a seismic paradigm shift, and veganism emerges as the guiding light towards a cleaner, revitalized lymphatic system. It's not merely a diet; it's a lifestyle that aligns with our evolutionary roots as fruitarians. Our anatomy, from our teeth to our digestive systems, hints at a design primed for the consumption of fruits. Embracing veganism isn't just a choice; it's a return to our natural state, a reconnection with the essence of our being.

Unlocking the Power of Fruits: Nature's Detox Elixir

At the very core of the vegan lifestyle lies an abundance of fruits, nature's most potent healers. These vibrant, living foods hold the key to unlocking your body's innate potential for cleansing and rejuvenation. Envision your plate as a canvas painted with the colors of nature's bounty – citrus fruits, berries, watermelon, mangoes – each bite an elixir that sweeps away toxins and ushers in vitality.

Fruits as Detox Powerhouses

Delve into the world of fruits, and you'll discover a myriad of natural compounds that act as detox powerhouses. Citrus fruits, laden with vitamin C, stimulate the production of glutathione, a key antioxidant that aids the liver in detoxification. Berries, rich in antioxidants, combat oxidative stress and assist in flushing out harmful substances. Watermelon, with its high water content, acts as a natural hydrator, supporting kidney function in expelling toxins. Mangoes, brimming with fiber, aid in digestion and promote regular bowel movements, a crucial aspect of detoxification.

Fruitarian Wisdom: Rediscovering Our Roots

Humans, in their primal state, were fruitarians. The anatomy of our teeth, the structure of our digestive systems, and our biological design all point to a diet rich in fruits. It's a return to the essence of our existence, a revival of the lifestyle that sustained our ancestors. By embracing the wisdom of fruitarianism, we reconnect with the harmony of nature and our bodies.

Fruitarians in History

Journey back in time, and you'll find that fruitarianism is deeply rooted in human history. Ancient civilizations, including the Essenes and ancient Greeks, recognized the vitality and health benefits of a fruit-based diet. Even renowned figures like Leonardo da Vinci and Pythagoras embraced fruitarian principles, acknowledging the profound connection between fruit consumption and optimal health.

Veganism and Lymphatic Cleansing: The Detox Symphony

Your lymphatic system, a network crucial for immune function and detoxification, finds unparalleled support in the vegan lifestyle. The absence of animal products alleviates the burden on this intricate system, allowing it to function optimally. A diet centered around fruits, with their high water content and natural enzymes, becomes the elixir that flushes out accumulated toxins, paving the way for renewed health.

Fruits and Lymphatic Health

Delving into the intricacies of the lymphatic system reveals that fruits play a crucial role in its optimal function. The high water content of fruits aids in lymphatic fluid circulation, preventing stagnation and promoting efficient toxin removal. Enzymes present in fruits support the breakdown of substances that may hinder lymphatic flow. Berries, in particular, with their antioxidant properties, assist in reducing inflammation and maintaining the health of lymph nodes.

The Healing Symphony of a Vegan Plate

Crafting your meals as a symphony of vibrant vegetables and fruits is not just a culinary choice – it's a healing ritual. Leafy greens, cruciferous vegetables, and the vivid spectrum of fruits harmonize to create a composition that resonates with your body's inherent rhythm. The antioxidants, phytochemicals, and fiber found in these plant-based wonders orchestrate a melody of health, cleansing, and rejuvenation.

The Role of Vegetables

While fruits take center stage, the supporting cast of vegetables adds a dynamic layer to the symphony. Leafy greens, like kale and spinach, offer a wealth of chlorophyll, known for its detoxifying properties. Cruciferous vegetables, such as broccoli and Brussels sprouts, contain compounds that support liver detoxification. The combination of fruits and vegetables creates a synergy that enhances the overall detoxifying effect.

Nourishment Beyond the Body: Earth-Friendly Detox

Veganism extends beyond physical nourishment; it encompasses the spirit and the planet. By choosing a plant-based path, you contribute to a sustainable, compassionate world. The benefits ripple beyond your well-being, reaching the very fabric of the Earth. It's a choice that echoes through the interconnected threads of life, fostering a harmonious relationship with the planet and all its inhabitants.

Embracing the Vegan Lifestyle: Practical Steps

Transitioning to a vegan lifestyle may seem daunting, but the journey is liberating. Start with gradual shifts – incorporate more fruits, vegetables, and plant-based proteins into your meals. Explore the vibrant world of plant-based recipes, savoring the diverse flavors nature offers. Allow your taste buds to dance to the symphony of plant-based delights, and witness the transformation unfold within.

The Transition Phase

Embark on the transition phase with an open mind and a willingness to explore new culinary horizons. Experiment with fruit-centric breakfasts, colorful salads, and plant-based protein sources. Embrace the wealth of resources available, from vegan cookbooks to online communities, where seasoned plant-based enthusiasts share their insights. This journey is not about restriction; it's about expanding your palate and embracing the abundance that nature provides.

A Future of Abundant Health: Veganism as the Ultimate Detox

As we conclude this expansive journey, envision a future where vibrant health is not an elusive dream but a tangible reality. The vegan lifestyle, rooted in fruitarian wisdom, becomes your compass. Your lymphatic system, cleansed and revitalized, propels you towards a life of boundless energy, mental clarity, and physical vitality.

Long-Term Benefits

Explore the long-term benefits of the vegan lifestyle, and you'll uncover a tapestry of health advantages. Reduced inflammation, enhanced immune function, and a lowered risk of chronic diseases become integral threads in this fabric of well-being. The vegan lifestyle is not a fleeting trend; it's a sustainable, lifelong commitment to optimal health.

As you embark on your detox journey, it's essential to recognize that various dietary approaches can contribute to the cleansing and revitalization of your body. Let's explore how you can achieve detoxification through different diet options, building upon the foundations discussed in this book.

Veganism: The Fruitful Path to Detox

The vegan lifestyle, with an emphasis on fruitarianism, stands as a powerful detoxifying agent. Fruits, with their high water content, fiber, and antioxidant properties, aid in flushing out toxins. A fruitarian approach involves consuming predominantly or exclusively fruits, harnessing their energy to cleanse and rejuvenate the body.

Action Steps:

- **Fruit Diversity:** Include a variety of fruits in your daily diet. Experiment with different colors, flavors, and textures.
- **Juicing:** Integrate fresh fruit juices or smoothies into your routine for a nutrient-packed detox boost.
- **Intermittent Fasting:** Consider incorporating intermittent fasting, allowing your digestive system to rest and enhance detox processes.

Plant-Based Whole Foods: A Balanced Approach

A plant-based whole foods diet, encompassing fruits, vegetables, legumes, and grains, aligns with detox principles. The fiber in whole foods aids in regular bowel movements, facilitating the removal of waste from your system. The diversity of plant-based nutrients supports overall health and detoxification.

Action Steps:

- **Colorful Plate:** Aim for a colorful plate by incorporating a variety of vegetables and fruits. The different hues signify diverse nutrients.
- **Hydration:** Ensure ample water intake to support the elimination of toxins through urine and sweat.
- **Herbal Teas:** Explore herbal teas known for their detoxifying properties, such as dandelion or ginger tea.

Functional Medicine and Personalized Detox Plans

Functional Medicine provides a personalized approach to detox, addressing the root causes of health issues. This includes assessing factors like genetics, lifestyle, and environment. Tailoring your diet based on Functional Medicine principles involves identifying specific food sensitivities and focusing on nutrient-dense, anti-inflammatory choices.

Action Steps:

- **Consult a Functional Medicine Practitioner:** Seek guidance from a Functional Medicine practitioner to assess your unique health profile.
- **Elimination Diets:** Experiment with elimination diets to identify foods that may contribute to inflammation or sensitivities specific to your own body.

- **Supplements:** Consider targeted supplements recommended by a healthcare professional to support detox pathways.

Intermittent Fasting: Time-Restricted Eating

Intermittent fasting involves cycling between periods of eating and fasting. This approach allows the body to enter a state of rest and repair during fasting periods, promoting cellular detoxification and renewal. It can be integrated into various dietary styles, including veganism and plant-based whole foods.

Action Steps:

- **Start Slow:** Begin with a gradual approach to intermittent fasting, such as a 12-hour overnight fast.
- **Adjust Timing:** Experiment with different fasting windows to find what suits your lifestyle and energy levels.
- **Monitor Energy Levels:** Listen to your body and adjust fasting patterns based on how you feel.

Mindful Eating: Detox for the Soul

Mindful eating goes beyond the realm of mere consumption; it extends to how you approach eating. Mindful eating involves savoring each bite, being present, and listening to your body's hunger and fullness cues. This approach can complement any dietary style, fostering a healthy relationship with food.

Action Steps:

- **Slow Down:** Practice eating slowly, savoring the flavors and textures of your meals. Counting the number of times you chew a single bite helps you to slow down and become aware and mindful of the eating process. Avoid distractions like a television or your cell cell phone during family dinners.

- **Gratitude Practice:** Cultivate a sense of gratitude for the nourishment your food provides to your body.
- **Emotional Awareness:** Be mindful of emotional eating triggers and strive to address them in non-food ways.

Crafting Your Detox Blueprint

In crafting your detox blueprint, consider the diverse array of dietary approaches discussed. Whether you lean towards a fruitarian vegan lifestyle, embrace plant-based whole foods, delve into the nuances of Functional Medicine, experiment with intermittent fasting, or practice mindful eating, the key is to find what resonates with you.

Remember, the journey to detox is not a rigid path but a dynamic exploration of what aligns with your preferences, health goals, and lifestyle. Combine elements from different approaches, experiment, and tailor your detox journey to become a unique expression of your well-being. As you navigate these diverse diets, may you discover the harmony that best nurtures your body, mind, and soul.

As you step forth into the future, remember that you are the protagonist of your own story. Your health and well-being deserve to be at the forefront. The pages of your journey are yet to be written, and each step you take moves you closer to your optimal state of health.

May this book, born from my experiences and driven by my

quest for health, empower you to embrace the possibilities of optimal health, and may it lead you on a path to lifelong vitality. It's time to continue your own journey, and I wish you every success as you embark on the next chapter of your life, with health as your guiding star.

Chapter 28: Recipes

H ere is a list of recipe options for the week in which you would have leftovers to freeze or eat the next day. Remember this is a lot of meals in a day, find what works best for you, 1 meal a day, 2 meals a day, or 3 meals a day with snacks. Listen to your body and it will provide your answers.

Monday
Breakfast
1/2 to a cup of organic oatmeal mix in favorite fruits blueberry, banana or apples and sprinkle in some cinnamon. Slice of avocado. Almond milk
Snack
organic peanut butter with banana or apple, collagen protein mix,
Lunch
6 oz of salmon, quinoa, olives, butternut squash
Snack
Salad with homemade dressing can add wild caught tuna, or other protein like chicken or chickpeas
Dinner
Some options for noodle are spaghetti squash, red lentil pasta,

chickpea pasta, rice noodles (no additives) with sausage and organic tomato sauce (look for extra virgin olive oil in the ingredients) no extra additives or just make your own tomato sauce if you have time and holds up great if you decide to freeze it.

Tuesday

Breakfast

2 to 3 scramble eggs, a little salt and pepper, avocado, homemade bread and home fries.

Snack

Fruit Salad (preferred organic) with your own favorite fruit

Lunch

Mac and cheese made from cashew cheese and rice pasta or other gluten free substitute. Think of some fermented foods like pickles, sauerkraut, olives and fermented cabbage.

Snack

Fruit smoothie

Dinner

Lamb and turkey kabob with Tzatziki sauce or tahini sauce with olives. Roasted Cinnamon Butternut squash and Roasted Asparagus. Cauliflower rice.

Wednesday

Breakfast

Almond and coconut flour pancakes with or without cocoa. Simmered blueberries or cinnamon applesauce. Kombucha to drink aims to find lower sugar kombucha.

Snack

Peanut butter protein cookie

Lunch

Yellow tuna salad with olives, purple onion and tartar sauce dressing. Quinoa
Snack
Yogurt or glass of kefir
Dinner
Cauliflower rice chicken bowl, with peppers, onions, lettuce, guacamole, salsa, small amount sour cream

Thursday
Breakfast
Oatmeal with banana, cashews, chia seeds, cinnamon, cocoa powder, almond milk, Greek yogurt with granola if one stomach can handle it. Piece of fruit
Snack
Vegetable smoothie and collagen protein
Lunch
Salmon, olives, sauerkraut, side salad with beets

Snack
Handful of nuts
Dinner
chicken shawarma, olives, lettuce wraps with Tzatziki sauce, roasted sweet potatoes and mushrooms.

Friday
Breakfast
shakshuka- classic Mediterranean breakfast, oatmeal and apple
Snack
Granola bar simple
Lunch

Halibut or walleye fish with olives, spaghetti squash and sauerkraut

Snack

Red pepper with guacamole

Dinner

Spaghetti squash and sausage spaghetti sauce (can make primavera sauce minus sausage)

Saturday

Breakfast

Buckwheat pancakes with mix berries some amount agave, Greek yogurt with mix berries blended with chia seeds and mix nuts cashews and almonds

Snack

Apple and peanut butter

Lunch

Salad with mixed vegetables and green and wild caught tuna and olives. Homemade dressing

Snack

Rice pudding

Dinner

Butter chicken with Baryina or white rice. Very nice Indian dish .

Sunday

Breakfast

Eggs with potatoes fries and avocados.

Snack

Smoothie

Lunch

Red lentil pasta with tomato sauce and side salad

Snack

Hummus with carrots and celery

Dinner

Zesty Cod with tomatoes and olives and potatoes fries and butternut squash

Green Smoothie or Juicer

Would include every day if you can, choose organic

1/2 of a cucumber

2 green apples

thumb size of ginger

1 full lemon include the rind, if there is wax, peel the lemon with a peeler

big handful of parsley

small handful of cilantro

small handful purple cabbage

2 tsp Cayenne pepper (this will not aggravate your gastrointestinal system but help aid in healing ulcers)

4 stalks celery

hand full of lettuce (preferably romaine or dandelion but any greens would work including sprouts. If you are concern about losing muscle consider adding alfalfa sprouts)

Rosemary Mustard Salmon

1 pound equal to 4 servings

1 lb 4 (4 ounce) salmon

1 .5 tablespoons of extra virgin olive oil

2 tablespoons Dijon mustard

1 teaspoon of rosemary fresh or dry

1 teaspoon thyme fresh or dry

½ teaspoon of salt preferred Himalayan salt or sea salt

½ teaspoon of black pepper
½ lemon

Directions

1. Preheat oven to 425 F
2. Use olive oil on aluminum foil and drizzle on fish
3. Combine the Dijon mustard, rosemary , thyme, salt, lemon and pepper and spread on fish, Place in gallon bag marinate in fridge overnight or 8 hr,
4. Cook Fish for 8 to 10 minutes

Tips if you choose to remove skin prior to cooking may have a chance of drying fish out but is quick and easier than pulling skin off when cooked. If you don't mind the skin, leave it on. Choose wild caught salmon preferred in the United States in Alaska. If one is choosing farmed salmon look for places like Norway instead of places like Chile has better farm practices but best bet is wild caught. I typically cook 2lbs of salmon or more at a time so I double the recipe and place in vacuum sealed bags and place in the freezer.

Lemon Oregano Fish (white fish, cod, walleye, halibut and etc.)
2lbs of fish of choice
2 lemons squeezed and ½ tablespoon of lemon zest from lemon peels
¾ cup of extra virgin olive oil
3 to 4 garlic cloves minced or chopped finely
2 tsp of dill weed
1.5 tsp of dried oregano

114

1 tsp black pepper

1 tsp of coriander

1 tsp of salt

I like to make this with green beans and onions and cherry tomatoes. If one has issues with seeds, use tomatoes and deseed it. If there are issues with onions, use leeks.

Directions

1. Preheat oven 425 F If cooking right away
2. In large bowl mix ingredients in sauce and place vegetables and coat and pull out with slotted spoon.
3. Used remaining sauce for fish and coat.
4. If choose to place in refrigerator overnight or 6 to 8 hours in gallon bag or cook right away.
5. Cook at 425 with fish and vegetables on the same cook pan. Cook fish for 12 to 15 minutes. You may need to cook green beans longer than the fish. Pull the rest of the food from the pan and leave green beans on the tray. Cook additional 10 to 15 minutes to desire texture.

Tips: Place green beans in separate bags if marinating in the refrigerator and by themselves on a baking tray to leave in the oven longer.

Chicken Shawarma

16 boneless, skinless chicken thighs

2 onions

1.5 lemon juice

½ cup of olive oil

1 Tbsp of ground cumin

1.5 Tbsp of turmeric powder
1.5 Tbsp of garlic powder
1.5 Tbsp Paprika
1.5 Tbsp ground coriander
¾ Tbsp ground clove
1 teaspoon of cayenne pepper
Salt
Olives

Serve with Romaine lettuce wraps/salad with Kalamata olives, deseeded plum tomatoes chopped up. Tahini sauce or Greek Tzatziki sauce

Directions

1. mix the cumin, turmeric, coriander, garlic powder, paprika and cloves in a bowl
2. pat chicken dry and season both sides with salt and slice into small bite size pieces
3. Place chicken in a large bowl, put in dry rub and coat chicken, then add lemon juice, onions and olives. Place in a gallon bag and place in the refrigerator for 6 hours or overnight for best taste. Don't have the time no problem cook it right away
4. Preheat oven 425 F. Pull chicken out of the refrigerator and let sit.
5. place chicken with onions on cooking pan(I usually cover pan with aluminum foil) and cook for 30 minutes
6. While cooking prepare sauce or do this step earlier for better tasting sauce and place in refrigerator

Greek Tzatziki Sauce

2 cups of greek yogurt, or sour cream, vegan yogurt

1 large cucumber grated, If one can't put the seeds outside and layers and chopped it up, don't use the seeded part.

1 large garlic clove mince

½ lemon juice

½ teaspoon dill optional

Salt and black pepper

Directions

1. Grated cucumber and add yogurt, garlic clove mince, lemon, and option dill
2. Add salt and black pepper for taste
3. cover place in fridge for 30 mins or overnight
4. The sauce can be kept in fridge for a week before it starts going bad

Tahini Sauce

½ cup tahini

3 garlic cloves minced

2 Tbsp of lemon juice

Pinch of ground Cumin

½ cup cold water for desire thickness add more or less

Directions

1. Combine garlic and lemon juice usually 10 minutes or more
2. Pour mixture with tahini, salt, pinch cumin and whisk
3. Pour in water for desire thickness

Lamb Kabobs (can make lamb and turkey or lamb and beef or just lamb)

2 lb of lamb (or substitute half with turkey or beef) 1 lb of lamb and 1 lb of turkey or beef

1 medium onion

2 cloves of garlic mince

½ cup of fresh parsley without the stems

¼ cup of cilantro

1 ½ tsp ground allspice

1 ½ tsp ground cardamom

½ tsp sumac or just zest from a lemon

½ tsp nutmeg

½ tsp paprika

½ tsp cayenne pepper

Salt and black pepper , I usually go with ½ tsp of each

Can serve with pita or top of salad or lettuce wraps

Can cook on grill of stove top

1. If grilling, soak 10 wooden skewers in water for 30 mins to 1 hour. Preheat the grill. If using stove top use ¼ cup pure olive oil can cook at higher temperature in a large pan
2. Chop onion, garlic, parsley and cilantro, can use a food processor if one chooses

3. Add in the meat of your choice, and all of the seasons allspice, cardamom, sumac or (lemon zest), nutmeg, paprika, cayenne pepper, salt and black pepper

4. Remove meat mixture and mold it on the wooden skewers for grilling or long hotdog shapes if using on stove top

5. Cook kabobs on medium heat , stove top for 10 minutes with rotating every 3 to 4 minutes, and same goes for the grill.

Tips
    Can serve with tahini sauce or Greek tzatziki sauce, lettuce wraps, salad, pitas (careful with additives and preservatives in store bought breads)

Almond Flour Banana Bread
    2 cups fine almond flour
    3 overripe bananas
    2 eggs or vegan options
    1 Tbsp. baking powder (I used cream of tartar and baking soda 2:1 ratio for substituted, doesn't have any additives that way)
    ½ tsp salt
    ½ pure vanilla extract
    3 dates medjool cooked (just place on stove top and cook with 2 cup water for 10 mins or till soft)
    1 tsp cinnamon
    ½ tsp nutmeg

Grease or line 9x5 loaf pan. I used coconut oil to grease the pan. Preheat oven 325 F and bake on center rack 50 to 55 mins. Let cool and go around the side with a knife, slice and enjoy the hold. Refrigerate well for a week or freeze extra time.
    Hummus
    15 oz. can chickpeas rinse off

Mash the chickpeas in bowl with a fork or use a food processor for smoother hummus

2 Tsp. olive oil

1 clove garlic mince

1 Tbsp of lemon juice

¼ tsp salt

1/8 ground cumin

Slice peppers for dipping and broccoli florets

Buckwheat Pancakes

1 ½ cup Greek yogurt

1 large egg

1 cup buckwheat flour

¾ cup of milk or coconut milk if avoiding milk

Mix in bowl cook on stove top for 2 min each side on low medium heat

Serve with fresh fruit strawberries or blueberries simmered on stove top for 5 minutes to provide a syrup consistency

Protein Peanut Butter Cookies

1 cup of organic peanut butter

1 cup coconut sugar or 6 cooked medjool dates, or half cup organic maple syrup

6 tablespoon of almond milk

2 tsp vanilla extract

1 cup of coconut flour

4 Tbsp. Of collagen peptides from vital proteins (optional)

1 tsp baking soda or cream of tartar with baking soda 2:1 ratio

Pinch of salt (sea salt or Himalayan salt)

Preheat the oven to 350 F, Mix ingredients in a bowl. Put in the refrigerator for 20 minutes. Use 1.5 Tbsp. scooper to roll in a ball and smash down with a fork.

Bake for 10 to 13 minutes allow to cool and enjoy

Rosemary French Fries
6 organic potatoes Yukon
Slices in wedges
1 tbsp of rosemary fresh or dry
3 to 4 tbsp extra virgin olive olive
Salt and pepper
Preheat the oven to 425 degrees, place season fries on a cooking sheet and cook for 50 mins. Allow to cool for 5 mins and enjoy.

Hot wings
4 lbs of chicken wings
Salt and pepper
Avocado oil
Sauce
2 tbsp Mc Ilhenny co Tabasco sauce
Kerrygold butter 4 tbsp
Pinch of cumin
Salt and black pepper
Take 4 lbs of chicken wings and place them dry with Paper towel. Place in the refrigerator overnight for best results for crispy wings uncovered. Pull out a place in a bowl mix salt pepper and avocado oil and place a rack on top of a cook sheet . Cook at 400 degrees for 45 mins. Allow to cool for 5 min

Sauce

On the stove top place in butter to melt and place in Tabasco sauce pinch of cumin and salt and pepper. Cook over medium heat for 5 mins. In a container with a lid, place in the wings and add the desired amount of sauce and shake. These wings will rock your world. You would think they are deep fried.

Spanish Rice

2 cups of organic brown

4 cups of water

Two tomatoes seeds taken out chopped

1 bell pepper chopped

1 onion chopped

1 tsp cayenne pepper

Salt

15.8 oz Can of chickpeas rinsed

Place onions, bell peppers on the stove on medium heat. Cook for 5 mins then add water. Place in cayenne pepper and add tomatoes, rice and chickpeas. Finish off with salt. Cook for 15 to 20 mins.

Granola Bar

3 cups rolled oats

1 cup sliced almonds (can soak in water overnight easier digestion)

1/2 cup honey

2 1/2 Tbsp organic peanut butter

1 1/2 tsp vanilla extract

1/2 cup of raisins

Preheat the oven 325 degrees, cook almonds and rolled oats for 10 mins. On the stove top melt honey, peanut butter, vanilla extract and raisins at the end. Pour over nuts on parchment paper. Cook for an additional 10 mins. Enjoy the granola.

Reference

Blumenthal, M., Goldberg, A., & Brinckmann, J. (Eds.). (2000). *Herbal Medicine: Expanded Commission E Monographs*. Integrative Medicine Communications.

Bown, D. (1995). *Encyclopedia of Herbs and Their Uses*. Dorling Kindersley.

Checallier, Andrew. *Encyclopedia of Medicinal Plants. 1996*

Clark, H. R. (1995). *The Cure for All Diseases*. New Century Press.

Clear, James. *Atomic Habits: An Easy & Proven Way to Build Good Habits & Break Bad Ones*. Penguin Random House, 2018.

Culpeper, N. (1826). *Culpeper's Complete Herbal, and English Physician wherein several hundred herbs are contained: with their names, virtues, places of growth, and time of flowering, collected and faithfuly described.*

Duke, J. A. (1985). *CRC Handbook of Medicinal Herbs* (1st ed.). CRC Press.

Hill, N. (1937). *Think and Grow Rich*. Random House.

Hoffmann, David. *Medical Herbalism: The Science and Practice of Herbal Medicine*. Healing Arts Press, 2003.

Kloss, J. (1992). *Back to Eden* (2nd ed.). Angell Press.

The institute for Functional Medicine (2020) Elimination Diet Comprehensive Guide, *https://p.widencdn.net/he7a5v/Elimnation-Diet*—-Comprehesive-Guide_v6

Morse R. (2004). The Detox Miracle Sourcebook: Raw Foods and Herbs for Complete Cellular Regeneration. Kalindi Press.

Williams, R. J. (1956). *Biochemical Individuality*. John Wiley & Sons.

Epilogue

These chapters serves as a bridge, a testament to the power of knowledge, persistence, and the right guidance in the pursuit of wellness. Detoxification isn't just a physical process; it's a mental and emotional journey of hope, setbacks, and triumphs.

As you embark on your own path of deep detoxification, remember that it's a journey of years, not just days or months. It's a testament to the strength and resilience of the human body.

www.ingramcontent.com/pod-product-compliance
Lightning Source LLC
Chambersburg PA
CBHW022100020426
42335CB00012B/765